USING PERSONAL JUDGEMENT in NURSING AND HEALTHCARE

USING PERSONAL JUDGEMENT IN NURSING AND HEALTHCARE

DAVID SEEDHOUSE & VANESSA PEUTHERER

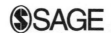

Los Angeles | London | New Delhi
Singapore | Washington DC | Melbourne

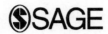

Los Angeles | London | New Delhi
Singapore | Washington DC | Melbourne

SAGE Publications Ltd
1 Oliver's Yard
55 City Road
London EC1Y 1SP

SAGE Publications Inc.
2455 Teller Road
Thousand Oaks, California 91320

SAGE Publications India Pvt Ltd
B 1/I 1 Mohan Cooperative Industrial Area
Mathura Road
New Delhi 110 044

SAGE Publications Asia-Pacific Pte Ltd
3 Church Street
#10-04 Samsung Hub
Singapore 049483

Editor: Alex Clabburn
Assistant editor: Jade Grogan
Production editor: Tanya Szwarnowska
Copyeditor: Clare Weaver
Proofreader: Jill Birch
Indexer: Silvia Benvenuto
Marketing manager: George Kimble
Cover design: Wendy Scott
Typeset by: C&M Digitals (P) Ltd, Chennai, India
Printed in the UK

Library of Congress Control Number: 2019955642

British Library Cataloguing in Publication data

A catalogue record for this book is available
from the British Library

ISBN 978-1-5264-5899-5
ISBN 978-1-5264-5900-8 (pbk)

CONTENTS

If you choose not to decide, you still have made a choice

Freewill, Rush

O, wad some Power the giftie gie us

To see oursels as others see us!

It wad frae monie a blunder free us,

An' foolish notion.

Robert Burns

We're not separate observers of an objective world. We're an inextricable part of it, connected to everything and everyone around us, past, present and future. Both in nursing and in life in general we have vastly more impact than we imagine.

David Seedhouse

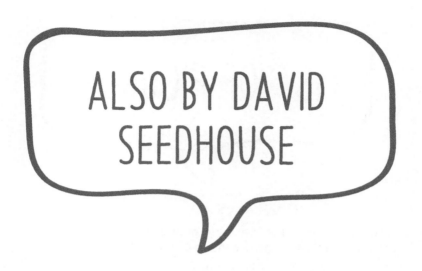

ALSO BY DAVID SEEDHOUSE

Health: The Foundations for Achievement, 1986, 2001

Ethics: The Heart of Health Care, 1988, 1998, 2009

Changing Ideas in Health Care (edited, with Alan Cribb), 1989

Liberating Medicine, 1991

Practical Medical Ethics (with Lisetta Lovvett), 1992

Fortress NHS: A Philosophical Review of the National Health Service, 1994

Reforming Health Care: The Philosophy and Practice of International Health Reform (edited), 1995

Health Promotion: Philosophy, Prejudice and Practice, 1997, 2003

Practical Nursing Philosophy: The Universal Ethical Code, 2000

Total Health Promotion: Mental Health, Rational Fields and the Quest for Autonomy, 2002

Values Based Decision-Making for the Caring Professions, 2006

Thoughtful Health Care, 2017

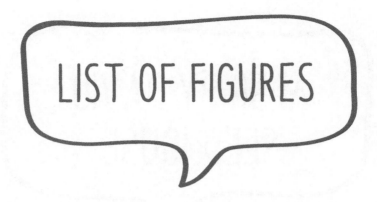

LIST OF FIGURES

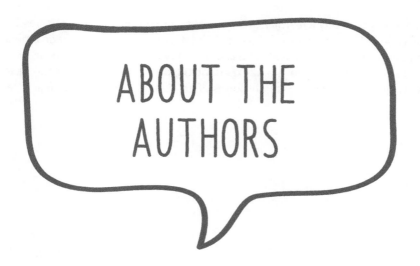

ABOUT THE AUTHORS

DAVID SEEDHOUSE is the creator of the Values Exchange – or 'social networking with brains' as he sometimes likes to call it: www.values-exchange.com. David's mission is to promote deep thinking and clear communication about the social issues that affect us all – by using both books and the internet for structured, tolerant democratic engagement.

The Values Exchange is used by universities, health services and schools in Australia, New Zealand and the UK. David currently runs the Values Exchange on a part-time basis and is Honorary Professor of Deliberative Practice in the School of Pharmacy at Aston University, UK.

David was Professor of Health and Social Ethics at Auckland University of Technology for eleven years and Professor of Health Care Analysis at Middlesex University, UK for three years. He was also founding editor of the international journal *Health Care Analysis*, which he edited for seven years.

David has written 16 other books including second and third editions. His most well-known are the bestselling *Health: The Foundations for Achievement, Ethics: The Heart of Health Care* and *Health Promotion: Philosophy, Prejudice and Practice*.

You may like to access David's LinkedIn profile to find out more: http://nz.linkedin.com/in/davidseedhouse

VANESSA PEUTHERER studied at the Royal Devon and Exeter School of Nursing. Now retired from active practice, she has long and varied experience in acute and elective adult hospital care, teaching and assessing in clinical practice, advanced life support and first line management. Vanessa also worked as a consultant on clinical negligence reviews and scrutiny panels and remains an active researcher.

Vanessa devised this book because she believes passionately in providing health professionals with adequate support and debriefing opportunities in order to retain an experienced, valued workforce.

Vanessa is currently a learning and development consultant for the Values Exchange and a writer of healthcare ethics scenarios for both pre- and post-registration programmes, both in universities and the NHS. She is a keen advocate of critical thinking, thoughtful healthcare, reflective practice and experiential learning through simulation exercises. Vanessa also enjoys creating various forms of art, forest walking and is an avid reader.

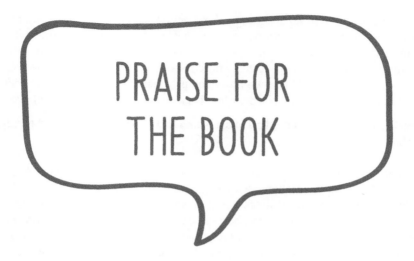

PRAISE FOR
THE BOOK

This book makes a valuable, innovative and practical contribution to the literature on decision-making and ethics in care. The book builds on philosopher David Seedhouse's substantial body of work in philosophy as applied to health and care. It is unusual in bringing together the experience of a philosopher and an expert nurse. The book focuses on 'personal judgement', underpinned by fast and slow thinking, and draws attention to the complex and multi-faceted nature of decision-making in care contexts. It provides an abundance of scenarios, frameworks and resources that will be helpful to students of health and social care. The book may also assist teachers as they help students negotiate challenging scenarios and respond to uncertainty and disagreements in care. Unusually, the book makes explicit different – and sometimes conflicting – reflections on particular decisions. This role modelling of different perspectives is likely to stimulate critical reflection and discussion regarding care scenarios. This book will complement the existing literature relating to decision-making and ethics in care.

Ann Gallagher, Professor of Ethics and Care, International Care Ethics Observatory, University of Surrey and Author of 'Slow Ethics and the Art of Care' Emerald 2020

A timely, well written book on decision making which I thoroughly recommend. A corrective to 'check box' culture and normative rule following.

Benny Goodman, Author, Independent Researcher and Scholar

David and Vanessa's reflections are worthwhile and enable the reader to understand potential perspectives which may differ from their own and therefore further opportunity to broaden considerations.

Claire Peers, Lecturer of Adult Nursing, University of Plymouth

I believe it is a timely book which serves as a useful resource for all health professionals in how we might cope with conflicts and issues that will inevitably arise in their future practice. This book and the well-considered scenarios cover a range of pertinent topics, the reflections by both are very thought provoking. They provide some very humane responses to different situations. David and Vanessa's reflections complement each other well and are really useful in offering different perspectives on the same scenarios. This sets the book apart as too often we have commentary from one person whose word then becomes unilateral. This does not reflect reality where people have their own unique voices. We live in an ambiguous world and we must equip students to cope in this environment. This book exposes us to this. I will be using this in my teaching of radiography students.

John McInerney, Lecturer of Medical Imaging and Radiation Sciences, Monash University, Australia

If computers could make all the decisions, we would not need human beings. A significant challenge in healthcare education is enabling students to find a balance between following the rules and algorithms of healthcare and creating a truly respectful and collaborative relationship with patients. What the authors do very well is re-frame this balancing act to show the importance of personal judgement, how this is influenced for better or worse by our inherent psychology, and most importantly how a conscious awareness of the processes can make healthcare practitioners more reflective and more effective decision-makers.

Mark Brennan, Deputy Head of Pharmacy & Reader in Healthcare Ethics and Law, Aston University

This book challenges the received wisdom of normative and inductive ethics and requires the reader to engage in ethical thinking utilising a wholly new paradigm which includes asking questions of oneself. I commend this book to any practitioner looking to understand ethical practice within modern healthcare.

Peter Ellis, Independent Nursing Educational Consultant and Writer

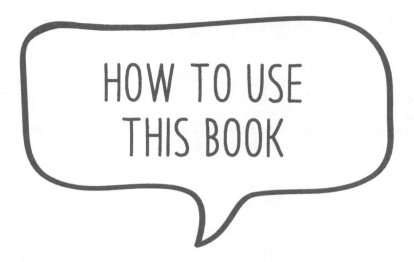

HOW TO USE THIS BOOK

This book clarifies decision-making in nursing and healthcare. It explains that personal judgement is essential in everyday practice, and offers realistic scenarios for personal reflection and group debate.

There are four main ways to use the book:

TO LEARN

- The contemporary context of nursing and healthcare decision-making
- Some common models and theories of decision-making in nursing and healthcare
- Different decision-making approaches you can apply to solve everyday problems of healthcare practice
- The nature and importance of personal judgement

TO TEACH

- Background theory
- Experiential learning and simulation
- Critical thinking
- Reflective practice
- Ethical deliberation
- Action learning sets
- Realistic, everyday nursing and healthcare problems where there are no obviously right answers, and where personal judgement is indispensable

TO PRACTISE PERSONAL JUDGEMENT

- The basic components of personal judgement are explained
- 43 everyday nursing and healthcare scenarios are described
- Readers are strongly encouraged to use the scenarios, plus whatever decision-making approaches they think most appropriate, to decide what to do in each
- Exercises to boost confidence in personal judgement are included. They can be used individually, in lectures, in small groups and in the workplace

TO BUILD SELF-AWARENESS

- How we make decisions as individuals is less predictable and affected by a far wider mix of influences than we typically believe
- To know and accept variability in ourselves and others is a vital skill if we are to achieve the best outcomes in healthcare and life in general

In order to maximise learning opportunities, each chapter includes simple aims and learning outcomes at the beginning, and reinforcing exercises at the end.

We use gender terms – he, she, him, her, etc. – interchangeably.

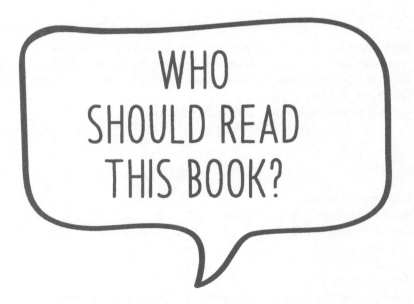

WHO SHOULD READ THIS BOOK?

This book is designed for nursing students and lecturers from first year undergraduate to postgraduate and advanced practitioner, as well as students and lecturers in any other clinical and allied health discipline. It is particularly effective in programmes on critical thinking, decision-making, reflective practice and ethics.

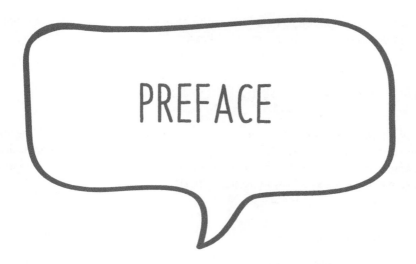

PREFACE

This book is a collaboration between a philosopher of health (David) and a retired nurse (Vanessa). Throughout our very different careers we were continually struck by the contrast between the 'official rule-based version' of healthcare practice and its messy, uncertain reality. As a practitioner, Vanessa felt restricted by the deluge of instructions, which came to dominate her natural sense of what it is to care for others creatively and compassionately. Rather than facilitate her autonomous, person-centred practice, she found that the rules tended to shift the focus of her nursing from the individual patient to the interests of the institution, and hampered her instinctive capacity to care responsively and humanely.

As a philosopher, standing outside health care looking in, David also found the bulging rule books troubling. Coming from an academic discipline where every term requires careful definition and justification, he found it hard to understand the merit of sweeping declarations – for example about acting in people's 'best interests' – which did not specifically explain what people's real-life 'best interests' actually are. Nor could he fathom the need for professional bodies to try to stipulate, with so many general clauses, how health professionals should and shouldn't behave. As a university lecturer for nearly 40 years, David taught thousands of students yet never had an official ethical code to follow. He merely tried to be kind, diligent and constructive. If health workers are intelligent, caring, responsible and well educated, do they really need to be told so extensively how to behave?

On discussing our experiences we came to the conclusion that healthcare has become imbalanced. We appreciate that it's a highly pressured environment where even the simplest mistakes can have massive consequences, and we understand that regulations are an obvious way to try to prevent or minimise damage. But in the process it seems to us that the essence of work for health – the personal, sensitive, human element – has been undermined.

This book is our attempt to explain the importance of this ubiquitous personal quality. We explore it practically – using everyday healthcare examples – and theoretically – with as much intellectual clarity as we can muster. We try to understand what it is, what it can and cannot do, and how it might best be employed to promote health. Our aim is to make a small contribution to help restore the balance between creative autonomy and standardised practice in nursing and healthcare.

HOW DID WE GET HERE?

As we contemplated writing this book together, we first tried to understand how present-day nursing and healthcare has come to regard decision-making. It's a complex area, and the danger of over-simplification is ever-present. However, we found the idea of a basic spectrum compelling as a 'way in' to the subject:

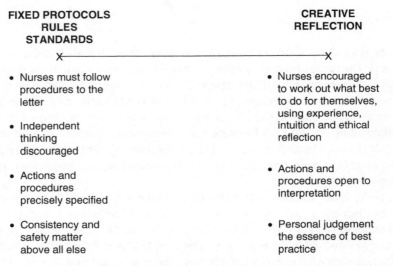

FIXED PROTOCOLS
RULES
STANDARDS

CREATIVE
REFLECTION

- Nurses must follow procedures to the letter

- Independent thinking discouraged

- Actions and procedures precisely specified

- Consistency and safety matter above all else

- Nurses encouraged to work out what best to do for themselves, using experience, intuition and ethical reflection

- Actions and procedures open to interpretation

- Personal judgement the essence of best practice

Figure 0.1   Spectrum 1. A Simple Representation of Two Poles of Contemporary Nursing and Healthcare Decision-Making

At the left, there are rules and standards, which, in an extreme case, could be applied with little if any thought. To the right, the professional is free to decide for herself what best to do: she may choose to follow a precise protocol or she may decide to do something quite innovative. At this end of the spectrum it's up to her.

Most nurse scholars agree that nurses ought to work as much as possible to the right of the spectrum, combining clinical expertise, evidence and patient preferences to make the most creative decisions (1). For example, Patricia Benner, a well-known nurse theorist, points to a 'perceptual skill' that grows with practice, enabling experienced nurses to grasp a patient's situation intuitively, through 'pattern recognition' (2). Other researchers have found that seasoned nurses develop the ability to anticipate events, which helps them be 'one step ahead' in patient care (3); while thoughtful nurses routinely confer with peers to try to work out the best solutions in difficult or unstructured circumstances (4).

The UK's official nursing body – the Nursing and Midwifery Council (**NMC**) – also encourages nurses to be independent problem solvers, even to the extent of challenging practice where they find it lacking (**5**). Yet at the same time, nursing decision-making models to the left of the spectrum – which advise step-by-step, uniform processes – are extensively recommended and taught. Nurses are expected to apply official protocols and ethical codes to the letter – both by their employers and their professional associations. And to the dismay of many health professionals, there are ever more forms to complete and check-boxes to tick (**6, 7**).

If we're right in thinking that the left pole of the spectrum has become disproportionately dominant, why and how has this come about? How did we get here?

WHY RULES?

There are very obvious reasons to have rules and standards. Individual health professionals must know best evidence in all areas of their work, demonstrate the competence to deliver accordingly, be able to understand and act upon complicated legislation, and wherever possible use validated clinical pathways and decision-making algorithms to decide what to do. Standards are designed to guarantee the minimum level of care an individual patient should expect to receive.

Seen more broadly, through the eyes of professional bodies and major healthcare organisations, the world of practice looks increasingly risky and, therefore, in need of cautious and effective management. There has been a recent series of scandals where possibly thousands of patients have been damaged or killed through poor standards of care (**8, 9**) and multiple official inquiries have made literally hundreds of recommendations for change and improvement (**10**). A good number of these recommendations refer to applying standards, for example:

- A code of conduct should be established for those working with elderly, and vulnerable patients.
- A common code of ethics and conduct, based on patient needs and public expectations, should be adopted by all senior managers in the NHS.
- Healthcare support workers should undergo consistent training, and should be regulated by a registration scheme.
- Hospitals should agree lists of 'fundamental standards' about patient safety, effectiveness and basic care.
- Standards should be created by the National Institute for Health and Clinical Excellence (**NICE**) policed by the Care Quality Commission (**CQC**).

Codes and standards are not only an attempt to increase safety and uniformity, they can also be used by practitioners and managers to improve specific practices. If for example, due to lack of resources, it's not possible to treat every patient with dignity all the time, citing a failure to follow an ethical code can be a powerful agent for change.

Beyond codes and mission statements, initiatives such as 'intentional rounding' (a mandatory hourly check on each patient regardless of their condition) and the 'friends and family test' ('would you be happy for your relatives to be treated in this hospital?') have been introduced to try to improve clinical outcomes and measure patient satisfaction (**11**). In addition, there's a relentless managerial drive to lower legal claims for negligence, which are a consequence of poor practice, cost the NHS £1.7 billion in 2017 and have a direct impact on what can be spent on frontline care (**12**).

THE LIMITS OF RULES

Rules, protocols and pathways are central to clinical practice. Teaching and delivering the most effective, evidence-based treatment is essential to the best and most consistent science-based healthcare, and is required and expected by law. Working 'according to the book' – whether it be prudent prescribing, effective clinical procedures or prompt and appropriate referral – is by far the most conspicuous part of modern healthcare.

Unfortunately, however, the high visibility and sheer volume of protocols has created a rule-based culture in which **every** part of healthcare – not just the clinical aspects – is considered equally amenable to step-by-step pathways and algorithms. But extending rules into areas of practice where more than one set might reasonably be applied – patient-centred care and health promotion, for instance – is quite a different matter from using best evidence to stipulate the **ideal** methodology for heart valve surgery. Consequently, in the interest of realism and balance, this book highlights the vast yet sparsely charted area of healthcare where the evidence is **not** definitive, where there are multiple viable options one could choose, and where personal judgement beyond protocols is simply indispensable.

WHERE RULES ARE NOT ENOUGH

The steady evolution of a standardised healthcare culture is easy to understand. But evolution does not always bring about the best results. There are limits beyond which it becomes counter-productive, and it can even collapse.

There are two main problems with an over-reliance on rules:

- If the rules are **imprecise** – as they are in every area where there's no absolute certainty, including clinical practice – they require interpretation if they are to be applied. When rules require interpretation, this interpretation must be beyond the rules themselves, since interpretation can be done only by people. For example, nurses are required to show that they value 'commitment' (**13**), but what they should be committed to is an open question, and has to be decided by human beings.
- Where the rules are **specific**, they soon contradict each other, because in the vast and complex healthcare world they are always created *ad hoc* and piecemeal, rather than according to a coherent overall plan.

Examples of **imprecision** are everywhere in official guidance documents. For example:

> Registered nurses (should) act in the best interests of people, putting them first
> and providing nursing care that is person-centred, safe and compassionate. (**14**)

In principle it's hard to disagree with this statement, but in actual practice defining the terms and then specifically deciding what to do can be a complex challenge. Hard choices have to be made, and there's no guarantee that the health professionals who must make them will concur. In fact, it's highly unlikely that they will. All 43 scenarios in this book demonstrate this phenomenon. We can all assent to putting patients first, but whenever patients disagree with each other (for example, about eating smelly food on the ward or about noise levels) or with you (for example, about their medications or when they should take meals or which staff members should care for them), a judgement beyond the guidelines and proficiencies is required.

Examples of **specific** contradictions are equally abundant. For example, in nursing, in addition to the many clauses in the Nursing and Midwifery Council (**NMC**) Code, there are currently six main standards, most of which have a range of sub- or associated standards, and all of which need to be read alongside other regulations and guidelines (**15, 16, 17, 18**).

When you put all these recommendations together, as is formally required of you as a professional, you inevitably find that they do not gel readily into practical strategies. For example, on the ward Vanessa was required to carry out 'intentional rounding'. Every hour in the day and every two hours at night she was instructed to visit each patient on her list to inquire about his comfort and needs, and record each intervention in a log. While there is definitely merit in this approach, at the same time she was also supposed to practise according to the **6Cs** (**13**), one of which is:

Compassion

> Compassion is how care is given through relationships based on empathy, respect
> and dignity – it can also be described as intelligent kindness, and is central to how
> people perceive their care.

However, it's impossible for any nurse to conform to contradictory rules at once. Being compassionate requires a specific, time-consuming focus on particular individuals (some need more compassion than others) and may well make it impossible to complete the intentional rounding process, caring for everyone in the same way, according to a rota.

Rules also tend to accumulate. New rules and standards do not always replace previous measures, and this can cause a snowball effect of confusing, conflicting – and at times overwhelming – bureaucratisation. Indeed, there are now so many rules it's impossible to abide by them all, however willing you are to do so. For example, the educational standard quoted below could mean pretty much anything you want it to, and if applied to the letter would be practically paralysing:

> 3.2 ensure that students experience the variety of practice expected of registered
> nurses to meet the holistic needs of people of all ages. (**19**)

Expecting teachers to offer students sufficient variety of practice to meet every patient's life needs is surely asking too much.

We can see and appreciate how much thought and effort the **NMC** has put into its standards and guidelines. These days almost all businesses and social institutions offer similar guidance, and the **NMC** has certainly put in more time and attention than most. Nevertheless, whatever organisation takes this quasi-legal approach, it simply won't be able to deliver the result it aspires to. This is just a fact of life. Sooner or later – and usually sooner – rules and guidelines are not enough, and people have to think for themselves, creating difference rather than uniformity as a result.

We do understand the pressures on healthcare institutions to deliver everything in line with a blueprint. And we can certainly see why more and more standards and more and more ethical codes can seem like a solution. But we do not agree that this is a sustainable answer, as we comprehensively explain in this book. Of course, people will carry on writing standards and rules – and these will continue to offer helpful general guidance – however, it's vital to recognise that these dictums scarcely touch the reality of daily health care, as our commonplace scenarios show.

Perhaps our most striking discovery in writing this book is how often and how quickly the rules fall away in everyday practice. It turns out that far from being only occasionally required to deal with unusual or exceptional circumstances, personal judgement is constantly and everywhere needed for effective, intelligent healthcare. Personal judgement is not an optional extra, or an occasional adjunct to rule-based practice. It truly is the human heart of healthcare (**20**).

In the end, anywhere other than at the clinical cutting edge, so many rules and standards are disadvantageous. If every aspect of nursing is taught as nothing more than a matter of following instructions and pathways, checking boxes and filling in forms, then on those many, inevitable occasions when only personal judgement will do, nurses will flounder and almost certainly be less safe and effective as a result.

THE CHALLENGE

As writers and thinkers, who wish to use our minds and experience to support and improve healthcare education and practice, we were most definitely aware that we faced a massive challenge in writing this book. We're operating in a rule-based culture that's advocated by every official body, is promoted in most texts for students, and is comprehensively validated in accredited health professional education. Yet despite its popularity, this culture fails to properly appreciate, or possibly is even afraid of, the free-thinking human factor.

Consequently, we decided that we must engage in an honest exploration of personal judgement, and that this must include pointing out the limitations of the present drive for more and more regulation and uniformity. Personal judgement happens constantly in healthcare. It often conflicts with or is quite different from the rules. But this does not mean that the rules and standards are unimportant, rather they are genuine attempts to encourage health professionals to be the best they can be – it's just that we feel that to achieve this we need standards AND we need self-awareness, creativity and personal engagement as well.

We're looking, we suppose, for the best of both worlds. Therefore, we encourage readers to research evidence-based practice (**EBP**), learn and apply the many professional standards if they wish, while reflecting on what they mean to them personally, using examples from experience wherever possible. And we also encourage readers to understand the power of personal judgement, to appreciate how essential to good practice it is, and to use this book's ideas and concrete examples to boost self-awareness, awareness of others, and awareness of life's complexities and differences.

There are encouraging signs that both shared standards AND deep personal reflection will increasingly be officially acknowledged, and will, therefore, form a vital part of future education and practice. For example, in 2019 the **NMC** began to recommend that:

> At the point of registration, the registered nurse will be able to:
>
> 1.8 demonstrate the knowledge, skills and ability to think critically when applying evidence and drawing on experience to make evidence informed decisions in all situations
>
> 1.10 demonstrate resilience and emotional intelligence and be capable of explaining the rationale that influences their judgments and decisions in routine, complex and challenging situations
>
> 1.14 provide and promote non-discriminatory, person-centred and sensitive care at all times, reflecting on people's values and beliefs, diverse backgrounds, cultural characteristics, language requirements, needs and preferences, taking account of any need for adjustments
>
> 1.17 take responsibility for continuous self-reflection, seeking and responding to support and feedback to develop their professional knowledge and skills
>
> 1.18 demonstrate the knowledge and confidence to contribute effectively and proactively in an interdisciplinary team (**21**)

While these requirements still lack exact guidance (how do you actually 'reflect on people's values and beliefs'? And if you find they are not the same as yours, can you really be 'non-discriminatory'?) we believe that this is as it should be. It would be impossible and pointless to write specific instructions for every set of circumstances, so we applaud these latest official attempts to encourage personal judgement. And we hope very much that our book will help connect these thought-promoting guidelines and attributes with the complexities and unknowables of everyday practice.

We are seeking to complement rather than dismiss official standards and decision-making approaches. We advocate using our modest **PSP** approach (explained in depth in **Chapter Four**) critically and open-mindedly, alongside and in combination with existing methods, tools and regulations. And where these latter become insufficient, then we encourage all health professionals to accept and embrace the need and opportunity to think and act personally – it happens all the time in any case.

A QUICK GUIDE TO THE BOOK'S KEY POINTS

As you read this book, it may be helpful to bear in mind a few key points:

- Caring for other people is impossible without personal involvement and judgement.
- Understanding this – and being confident in your own personal judgement – is essential if the best healthcare is to be given.
- Most decision-making happens unconsciously and almost instantly.
- When we make decisions we make them personally.
- We bring many parts of ourselves to each decision – our history, our personalities, our education, our beliefs, our biases, our fears, our optimism, and much more.
- Circumstances tend to change us, just as much as we change them. We are not wholly in charge of our decision-making.
- It may seem paradoxical to say that judgement is personal and at the same time not fully under our control as individuals, but this is the reality. We are unique individuals who mix uniquely with our circumstances – this is evidenced as soon as you start to think about what you would do in any of the scenarios we present throughout this book. You decide as you, but you are not immune from the changeable influences that make you the person you are at the moment you decide, nor are you a detached observer. When we view external circumstances – other people, problems to be solved, things that need to improve – we combine ourselves with these circumstances to create a unique reality (we call this reality a 'situation' – we create situations as we become personally involved with circumstances).
- Most decision-making takes place without the use of rules and guidelines.
- While much decision-making is invisible to us – and we cannot even be sure that the retrospective reasons we give were the real reasons behind our judgements – we can always try to improve it, with awareness and practice.

In order to improve personal judgement:

- It is helpful to be as aware as possible of the forces and biases that make us who we are at any moment.
- While much decision-making is unconscious, when there's time to reflect either in advance or retrospect it's important to understand your decision-making as much as you can.

In advance, look at what you are bringing to the judgement. What biases do you have? How are the circumstances affecting you? What are you feeling that others you know might not be feeling? In retrospect, ask: why did I decide that way? What did I bring to the decision? How was I influenced by what I encountered? What did others bring? How were they influenced? How different from theirs was the reality I created when I considered the circumstances?

- It is also helpful to observe ourselves in the process of decision-making, if we can. What is happening to us as we are choosing? How much is logical and how much is something more mysterious? How much is less than 'perfectly rational'? How much can we truly know?

- It is helpful to be self-critical.
- It is helpful to ask others what we could have done better and what we might do better next time.
- It is extremely helpful to practise on case studies and simulations – like the many we present in **Chapters Five, Six and Seven**. The more you practise the stronger your personal judgement will become.
- Finally, it is necessary to accept that there is a limit to how much we can even know ourselves.

We are aware that we make many of these points more than once in the book. We confess that we were unable to avoid some repetition simply because so much in this area is interrelated. Nonetheless, we feel this is helpful and justified (though ultimately this is for the reader to judge). Our reasons are:

- The book's message is different from and often conflicts with the official, received wisdom of the era, and so bears emphasis.
- Much of what we say is not intuitive and may therefore take some reinforcing.
- We approach our investigation of personal judgement from a variety of angles, but in the end cannot help but arrive at consistent conclusions.
- We expect that many readers will prefer to dip in and out of the book rather than read it all at once (it's not a short book after all).
- Each chapter is designed to be studied separately, as a self-contained read. It matters little where you start and end your reading.

Overall, the book is intended to help you use personal judgement in healthcare as sensitively and effectively as possible. We hope that reading it will assist you to gain confidence in your own decision-making and empower you to justify yourself as an autonomous practitioner who must deal with innumerable uncertainties in your daily work.

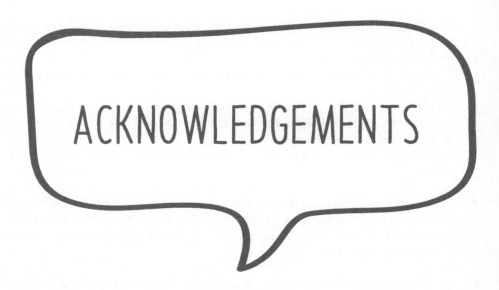

ACKNOWLEDGEMENTS

First, we would both like to acknowledge the support, professionalism and enthusiasm of the SAGE editorial team.

David would like to offer thanks to colleagues at Aston University whose faith in his teaching, writing and philosophy has been very important to him both professionally and personally. He would also like to say how fortunate he has been to work with Vanessa. It has been a privilege to be able to work with a retired nurse of such insight and integrity. Her rich, gritty scenarios reflect a reality of nursing and healthcare beyond his own experience, and pay testament to her powers of observation, and her kindness. We both hope we have achieved a helpful balance between the philosophical and practical investigation of personal judgement, and that this book will make a useful contribution to teaching and practice.

Vanessa would like to thank the many health professionals who have engaged with her scenarios on the Values Exchange. Their comments and feedback on several of the practice scenarios we use in this book have proved invaluable. Special thanks are also due to the employees of Nottinghamshire Healthcare NHS Foundation Trust, and many health professional students (pre and post grad.) at Coventry University, Lincoln University and Kingston University. Vanessa is particularly grateful to student nurse Katarina Gerhatova for sharing the practice scenario we adapted as 'The Woman and the Dog' and student nurse Murad Altanay for sharing the scenario which became 'Compassion for All?'

Vanessa thanks David for his relentless drive and passion for this writing collaboration, for running with the initial idea for a book of real-life scenarios for experiential learning, and for working so hard to make it a reality. She would also like to thank him for his belief in her nursing and healthcare knowledge and her strong intuition, which arises from it. David's philosophy of health is as close as any one will ever get to her own, and is something she deeply respects and endorses.

Finally, Vanessa would like to thank her extended family and friends for their encouragement, especially her dear friend Louise Underhill (RN) for her constant belief and unwavering support, and above all her teenage sons Zak and James for their patience while this work took her away from them.

All the errors and limitations in this book are, of course, our own.

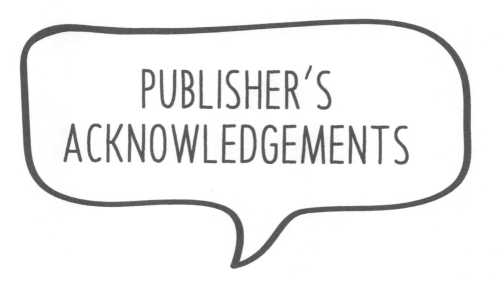

PUBLISHER'S ACKNOWLEDGEMENTS

The publishers would also like to thank the academic reviewers who provided invaluable feedback on the proposal for the book and draft material, helping to shape the book into a comprehensive resource for students.

Special thanks to:

Naim Abdulmohdi, Anglia Ruskin University

Beryl Cooledge, Bangor University

Peter Ellis, Independent Consultant

Jane James, Swansea University

Claire Peers, Plymouth University

CHAPTER 1
INTRODUCING PERSONAL JUDGEMENT

AIMS

This chapter has the following aims:

1) To explain how little is known about the moment of human decision-making
2) To introduce 'fast and slow thinking' – a well-known concept in psychology
3) To offer brief and simple models of nursing decision-making
4) To describe the wide gulf between these nursing models and the reality of human decision-making
5) To give examples of commonplace daily life and healthcare scenarios beyond the rules, where there are no clear-cut, right answers
6) To offer a simple definition of personal judgement and briefly discuss its implications
7) To encourage readers to see past generalisations and begin to appreciate the complexity of even apparently simple judgements

LEARNING OUTCOMES

When you have read and worked through this chapter you should be able to:

1) Appreciate and be able to explain, at an introductory level, the complexities of even the most everyday decision-making
2) Give your own examples of daily life and healthcare scenarios where there are no obviously right answers
3) Be able to explain and demonstrate why the need for personal judgement cannot be eliminated by nursing and healthcare models

WHAT IS PERSONAL JUDGEMENT?

The purpose of this book is to help nursing and health professional students and teachers better understand and use personal judgement. In order to do this it is obviously necessary to explore the nature of personal judgement, examine circumstances where it is needed, think about what happens when it occurs and – if possible – try to define patterns, draw meaningful conclusions and offer advice to those who wish to improve their decision-making. Frustratingly, however, this is far from straightforward. It would be foolish to attempt to say: 'this is how you should make good judgements' or 'this is a good judgement and this is a bad one' or 'we advise you to make this type of judgement and not that type'. As we shall see, decision-making is just too rich and complex to pin down in this way. The best we can do is try to clarify what personal judgement involves in general so that when we make a judgement we at least have some awareness of what's going on inside us, inside others involved, and how the interaction between ourselves and the external world affects what we choose.

Human decision-making – which is simply another term for personal judgement – remains a largely mysterious process. Despite millennia of human curiosity about it no one – not even the most astute and well-informed researcher – completely understands how people decide.

Psychologists know an enormous amount about how most of us make most decisions; however, it's impossible to predict specifically how any given person will choose in any given circumstances, simply because making a judgement is so complex. For example, there's a well-known phenomenon in psychology called 'the bystander effect', where people are less likely to help a person in distress the more people there are present.

> The bystander effect was first demonstrated and popularized in the laboratory by social psychologists John M. Darley and Bibb Latané in 1968 after they became interested in the topic following the murder of Kitty Genovese in 1964. These researchers launched a series of experiments that resulted in one of the strongest and most replicable effects in social psychology. In a typical experiment, the participant is either alone or among a group of other participants or confederates. An emergency situation is staged and researchers measure how long it takes the participants to intervene, if they intervene. These experiments have found that the presence of others inhibits helping, often by a large margin …. For example … [in one] experiment around a woman in distress …. 70 percent of the people alone called out or went to help the woman after they believed she had fallen and was hurt, but when there were other people in the room only 40 percent offered help. (**22**)

There are several illuminating videos about this phenomenon available on the internet (**23, 24**). But what is most interesting is that of the people referred to in the quote above, it's impossible to say beforehand who will be in the 40 per cent who will help and who will not – there are too many complex variables involved to tell. It's also not at all certain that if an individual intervenes in one situation she will, therefore, intervene in a similar one.

We can rationalise our judgements in retrospect but that may not be how we actually decided at the time. Sometimes we just don't know why we made the choice we did. Sometimes we surprise ourselves: 'I changed my mind at the last minute', 'maybe it's not such a good idea after all', 'I have no idea why I did that'. Sometimes the only certainty is that we, personally, made a choice – and next time we might make a different one – we just don't know:

> The mystery of how we make decisions – how Tom Brady [an American football quarterback] chooses where to throw the ball – is one of the oldest mysteries of the mind. Even though we are defined by our decisions, we are often completely unaware of what's happening inside our heads during the decision-making process. You can't explain why you bought the box of Honey Nut Cheerios, or stopped at the yellow traffic light, or threw the football to Troy Brown. On the evaluation sheets of NFL scores, decision-making is listed in the category Intangibles. It's one of the most important qualities in a quarterback, yet nobody knows what it is. (**25**)

Astonishingly, nearly a century of sustained scientific research has told us more about what we don't know than what we do. According to Kenneth Hammond, an academic who devoted his career to the subject:

... (1) human cognition is not under our control, (2) we are not aware of our judgement and decision processes and (3) our reports of those processes are not to be
trusted ... (**26**)

This is quite something. We cannot govern our thoughts, they occur to us unbidden. Unless
we make a determined effort to understand ourselves, we're oblivious to the ways we
make decisions. And as soon as we stop reflecting on our judgements, we revert to making
decisions without thinking about the process at all. What's more – if anybody asks us – the
way we believe we make our judgements is usually at odds with what the science tells us.

We are, however, able to explore some basic decision-making models in the
contemporary nursing and healthcare literature, look at examples of where personal
judgement is necessary (i.e. all the time and everywhere), and consider whether or not
the models help explain and improve personal judgement (they don't).

FAST AND SLOW THINKING

For our purposes in this book, and for the sake of simplicity, we will consider only two
general ways of making decisions:

FAST THINKING

Fast thinking is making decisions rapidly or even instantly, without being conscious of
the process at the time (**27**).

According to Nobel Prize-winning psychologist Daniel Kahneman, examples of fast
thinking, or System 1 as he calls it, are:

- determining that an object is at a greater distance than another
- displaying disgust when seeing a gruesome image
- solving 2 + 2 = ?
- reading text on a billboard
- driving a car on an empty road.

The defining characteristics of fast thinking are:

- unconscious, automatic, effortless
- without self-awareness or control – 'what you see is all there is'
- assesses the situation, delivers updates
- makes up 97% of all our thinking.

Fast thinking can be useful:

- when there is little or no time to reflect
- where experience is needed quickly, without the time for explicit calculation
- for life's constant stream of decisions.

SLOW THINKING

Slow thinking is making decisions deliberately and reflectively, either processing the decision according to rules and structures or through careful balancing of the pros and cons.

Kahneman's examples (he calls slow thinking System 2) include:

- bracing yourself before the start of a sprint
- digging into your memory to recognise a sound
- determining the appropriateness of a particular behaviour in a social setting
- determining the price/quality ratio of two washing machines
- determining the validity of a complex logical reasoning
- solving 17 × 24.

The defining characteristics of slow thinking are:

- deliberate and conscious, effortful, controlled mental process, rational thinking, infrequent, logical, calculating
- with self-awareness, analytical and sceptical
- seeks new/missing information, makes overt decisions
- constitutes 3% of human deliberation.

Slow thinking can be useful:

- when there is time to think before you need to choose
- in retrospect
- when there are 'large decisions' to be made. For example, restructuring a hospital or changing recruitment policies in a business.

It is of little or no use in everyday healthcare situations where the nurse or other health professional must think on his or her feet (i.e. in the great majority of decisions).

WE DON'T THINK IN THE WAYS WE THINK WE DO

This quite striking idea informs part of our theorising. It sits underneath our idea of **PSP**, which we explain in detail in **Chapter Four**. In essence, when we make decisions we bring everything about us as **persons** (the first **P**) – our personalities, our experiences, our values and preferences, our biological make-up – to a unique set of circumstances. As we decide – consciously or unconsciously – our unique selves combine with the circumstances in ways we can barely comprehend, to create **situations** (the **S**). Then, before we do anything a **plan** (the second **P**) is formed. If we are aware of this process then we can examine the plan. However, according to the science, in the vast majority of circumstances in which choice is required, nurses and other health professionals do not make conscious decisions according to official regulations, and then act. Rather they have a 'gut reaction' and act on that, without overt thought. Only for very complex or controversial choices where there is time to think, or in retrospect if they need to, do they refer to external regulations.

Official decision-making models and standards are based on the assumption that they will be used to guide and inform decisions **prior to** the decision itself, but this is not how things actually work. Vanessa occasionally used the **NMC Code (28)** to justify her decisions to others, but she never used it actually to decide. She made her own judgement, often quite spontaneously, and only then checked out to see if her decision was the best thing to do. She decided first and then considered, not the other way around.

The unavoidable conclusion is that models, competencies and codes are of limited use in real life. They provide a general map of good practice, and may help us reflect in retrospect. They can also be useful discussion points in classrooms, but they are only barely related to real life decision-making (see our discussion of 'the four principles' in **Chapter Two** for example). The science very clearly supports this conclusion **(29)**.

Importantly, this means that the conscientious nurse who deliberates about every practical choice carefully, weighing up the pros and cons 'according to the book', and only then decides, is a mirage. This is recognised in some nursing literature, for example:

> Decision-making models offer analytical tools which can be combined to provide useful insights [but] ... in the real world, most of our decisions are made unconsciously in our mind. **(30)**

The fact that we mostly think in ways it is hard to comprehend does not invalidate decision-making models, which are widely taught in nursing and healthcare. But it does mean that they are of only limited use, and are often irrelevant. It might even be argued that academic theorising and modelling is detrimental to practical decision-making, because it obscures the real picture. Nevertheless, it may be helpful to offer a simple list of some popular models in nursing.

SPECIFIC MODELS OF NURSING DECISION-MAKING

The brief list of nursing decision-making models below might be said to run roughly left to right along **Spectrum 1** (introduced in the **Preface**) though precisely where each fits is debatable:

- Fixed protocols and rules
- Clinical pathways
- Decision trees
- The nursing process
- The general decision-making model
- Holistic models

FIXED PROTOCOLS AND RULES — DEFINITELY SLOW THINKING

Decision-making protocols are widely referenced in the literature. Here's a rather extreme example:

1. Is the activity consistent with the Nursing Practice Act (NPA), Board Rules, and Board Position Statements and/or Guidelines?

        Yes – Continue   **No – STOP**

2. Is the activity appropriately authorized by valid order/protocol and in accordance with established policies and procedures?

        Yes – Continue   **No – STOP**

3. Is the act supported by either research reported in nursing and health-related literature or in scope of practice statements by national nursing organisations?

        Yes – Continue   **No – STOP**

4. Do you possess the required knowledge and have you demonstrated the competency required to carry out this activity safely?

        Yes – Continue   **No – STOP**

5. Would a reasonable and prudent nurse perform this activity in this setting?

        Yes – Continue   **No – STOP**

6. Are you prepared to assume accountability for the provision of safe care and the outcome of the care rendered?

        Yes – Perform the Activity   **No – STOP**

Figure 1.1   A Rule-Based Decision-Making Protocol (**31**)

The 'fixed protocol' model is sometimes also referred to as the 'information-processing model' which advises nurses to 'follow a (standard) set of procedures (of) cue acquisition, hypothesis generation, cue interpretation, and hypothesis evaluation', in clinical practice (**32**):

> The information-processing model is a ... scientific approach to making decisions ... [it has] four major stages [which are] gathering preliminary clinical information about the patient, generating tentative hypotheses about the patient's condition, interpreting the initially registered cues in light of the tentative hypotheses, and weighing the decision alternatives before choosing the one that fits best in light of the evidence collected. (**33**)

Following standard steps has obvious value in decision-making but it does not abolish the need for personal judgement. For example, the instruction 'weigh the decision alternatives before choosing the one that fits best' may sound straightforward yet, as we shall see, its apparent simplicity hides a complex mass of processes and personal choices.

CLINICAL PATHWAYS — SLOW AND STEADY THINKING

Clinical pathways are variously labelled as: care maps, care pathways, critical pathways, integrated care pathways, protocols and guidelines **(34)**. But whatever their name, they too set out generally favoured steps (not always in the same order) for managing clinical activities, for example:

> A critical pathway is appropriate after the acute phase of stroke care to outline best practice recommendations and highlight vital steps so nothing is forgotten, such as swallow evaluations, physical and occupational therapy evaluations, safety precautions, discharge planning, and patient education. This is where the multidisciplinary team collaborates, using critical pathway guidelines to develop an individualized care plan based on sound research and data to improve safety and outcomes. **(35)**

DECISION TREES — CAN BE COMPLEX, SLOW THINKING

Decision trees can be simple or enormously complex, if there are many variables to consider. However complex they are, they are nevertheless subject to personal judgement (the decision to use a decision tree is a judgement beyond the tree itself, as is how to weigh the pros and cons expressed within it). Figure 1.2 shows a simple decision tree.

THE NURSING PROCESS — STEP-BY-STEP SLOW THINKING

A further oft-cited step-by-step model is known as 'the nursing process':

The 5 Steps of the Nursing Process

The nursing process is a scientific method used by nurses to ensure the quality of patient care. This approach can be broken down into five separate steps.

Assessment Phase

The first step of the nursing process is assessment. During this phase, the nurse gathers information about a patient's psychological, physiological, sociological, and spiritual status ...

Diagnosing Phase

The diagnosing phase involves a nurse making an educated judgement about a potential or actual health problem with a patient. Multiple diagnoses are sometimes made for a single patient. These assessments not only include an actual description of the problem (e.g. sleep deprivation) but also whether or not a patient is at risk of developing further problems ...

Planning Phase

Once a patient and nurse agree on the diagnoses, a plan of action can be developed ...

Implementing Phase

The implementing (sic) phase is where the nurse follows through on the decided plan of action. This plan is specific to each patient and focuses on achievable outcomes ...

Evaluation Phase

Once all nursing intervention actions have taken place, the nurse completes an evaluation to determine which of the goals for patient wellness have been met ...

All nurses must be familiar with the steps of the nursing process. If you're planning on studying to become a nurse, be prepared to use these phases everyday in your new career. (**36, 37**)

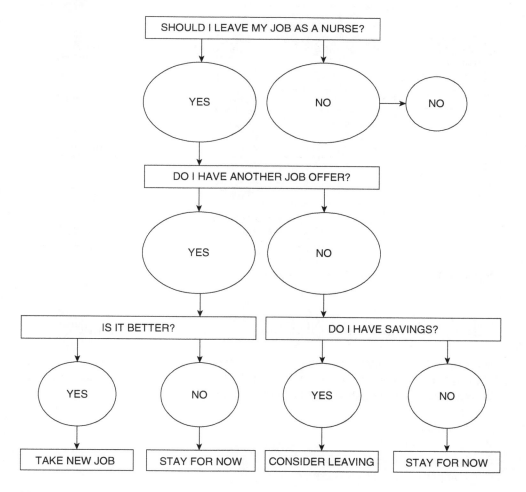

Figure 1.2   A Very Simple Decision Tree

Clinical pathways, decision-making protocols and the nursing process are basically the same idea with different names. Most nursing models are simply flow charts of one kind or another, designed to help organise care in logical progression, though some nurse commentators do find this linear approach problematic (**38**).

Seen in flow chart form in Figure 1.3, the models translate into this type of diagram, which, we have to say, do not always make matters any clearer.

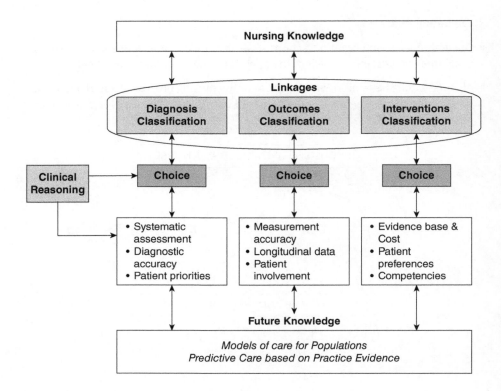

Figure 1.3   A Flow Chart Decision-Making Model (**39**)

GENERAL DECISION-MAKING MODEL — MORE SLOW THINKING

Most models in the literature refer to clinical tasks, but the same format may also be applied to more general decision-making, of the type we illustrate in our scenarios. For example, here is a straightforward suggestion of our own:

1. Identify the problem
2. Gather evidence
3. List ways to solve the problem
4. Compare and evaluate these

5. Choose the best option
6. Take action accordingly
7. Review the process in case it happens again

Note that items 1 and 2 must work in tandem.

HOLISTIC MODELS — SLOW THINKING, BUT MAY BE FAST IF INTUITION IS USED

At the right pole of **Spectrum 1** the literature refers to a '… humanistic-intuitive approach' which emphasises personal, emotional and contextual elements in decision-making, where nurses become increasingly intuitive decision-makers as their experience and knowledge develops **(40)**.

'Reflective practice', shown in Figure 1.4, is one example at this pole. The idea is that the more you reflect the better your intuitions will be.

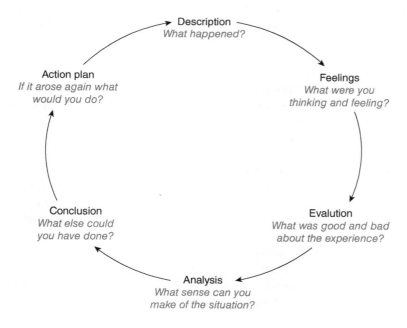

Description
What happened?

Feelings
*What were you
thinking and feeling?*

Evalution
*What was good and bad
about the experience?*

Analysis
*What sense can you
make of the situation?*

Conclusion
*What else could
you have done?*

Action plan
*If it arose again what
would you do?*

Figure 1.4   Gibbs' Reflective Cycle (**43**)

The most important feature of reflective practice is that it's personal. Unlike the more formal, objective protocols, it asks **you** – a unique individual – to think about what happened, from your point of view.

The idea that nursing is essentially personal has been elaborated by multiple nurse theorists, who tend to take keywords and develop a theory around them (**41**):

Caring in nursing is a holistic concept made apparent in nursing practice as a virtue through nurses' actions and attitudes, which are reflected by the deep knowledge they have of themselves as committed caregivers. (**42**)

Most holistic theories elaborate 'enabling concepts', like 'advocacy', 'respect', 'dignity' and 'caring', for example:

To care for another person … is to help him grow and actualise himself. Consider, for example, a father caring for his child. He respects the child as existing in his own right and as striving to grow. He feels needed by the child and helps him grow by responding to his need to grow. Caring is the antithesis of simply using the other person to satisfy one's own needs. (**44**)

And:

We are human beings, our patients or clients are human beings, and it is this commonality that should form the basis of the relationship between us. (**45**)

And:

[Advocacy] is the effort to help persons become clear about what they want to do, by helping them discern and clarify their values in the situation, and on the basis of that self-examination, to reach decisions which express their reaffirmed, perhaps recreated, complex of values. (**46**)

These concepts are clearly more personal and engaged with others than the guidelines to the left of the spectrum, but they too leave a great deal open to interpretation. Most people would surely agree that caring for someone is the opposite of using them, that nurses and patients are human beings, and that it can be a good thing to help patients work out what they want to do. But this advice is useless in circumstances where there's disagreement between carers and patients about what's best, or where there's competition between patients for resources. In these cases, deeper judgements are required.

Inescapably, whenever we wish to care for someone, in practice we face a question which forces us beyond generalisation: how should I care for **this** person in **these** circumstances?

OTHER NURSING MODELS

There are many other nursing models that are indirectly related to decision-making, but offer only basic or routine suggestions for daily care. For example, the Roper-Logan-Tierney 'activities of daily living' model of nursing (**47**).

A DISCONNECTION BETWEEN MODELS AND REALITY

Despite the best intentions of their authors, none of the models offer clear-cut help in real-life nursing circumstances. They may provide starting points, but apart from the very specific 'yes–no', 'proceed–don't proceed' protocols – which could just as well be undertaken by robots – the models offer general suggestions only. They leave the human, social elements open to the widest reading, and barely connect with the ways in which choosing and reflection actually happens.

All models (including the **PSP** model we offer in **Chapter Four**) are necessarily simplifications of reality. In order to represent the world in the most straightforward way they compartmentalise and separate the processes involved artificially. For example, in Gibbs' model, 'what were you thinking and feeling' is not actually separate from 'what sense can you make of the situation' but in the model it's presented as if it is (in fact your thinking and feeling has to be part of your sense-making).

By simplifying, models and theories leave most of the important questions unanswered. For example, is your evaluation of a situation the same as everyone else's, or is it different in significant ways? And if it is, in what ways is it different and how might these be explored? How do you actually involve patients in decision-making? Can they be equal partners or is this impossible, given the different backgrounds and knowledge of the carers and the recipients? What do you do if your helping a person clarify her values leads her to make what you consider to be a disastrous choice?

The truth is there are no standard procedures, rules or guiding theories for the great majority of decisions nurses have to make. Most aspects of nurses' daily working lives have no pre-set procedures at all.

REAL-LIFE DECISION-MAKING

Now let's look at some simple real-life situations to see how much the models help us. First, let's consider an elementary social example anyone can identify with:

EXAMPLE 1.1: THE TUNA QUICHE

You've been invited for lunch to a friend's house. You're vegetarian and have clearly explained this to your friend. Unfortunately, as it turns out, your friend is not entirely sure what 'vegetarian' means. You're at the lunch table now. It's loaded with bread and an appetising salad. Your host enters with a steaming hot quiche, which she proudly places centre-stage. You thank her, but look at the quiche suspiciously. She says, 'I don't usually do vegetarian but when I do this is my favourite.' You take a slice. You can see it has flakes in it that are unmistakably tuna. What's more, you look toward the open kitchen door and can see, on the counter, a large, opened can of best-quality tuna.

What do you do?

You may well think fast, and just react, deciding instantly or you could stall and start slow thinking instead. If so, there are rules and strategies you could apply to decide what to do. However, just as in nursing and all other professional life, these strategies do not choose themselves: **you** have to choose them. In the case of the tuna quiche there are various options open to you: tell the truth and refuse the quiche, eat it and don't say anything, eat the quiche but leave the tuna, say you feel sick, say you're allergic to seafood, pretend you have an urgent phone call – there are many alternatives. But which one you choose is always up to you, personally.

We constantly run into situations where there are no norms. Choosing what to say to people close to us (should I raise this difficult issue now, or avoid it?), behaving with work colleagues (should I take morning tea in the staff room or stay working at my desk?), reacting to others (I think this shop assistant is being unkind, should I challenge her?), controlling or not controlling one's emotions (that driver pulled right out in front of me – should I blow my horn and make a gesture or should I stay calm?). Every day and everywhere there are either no rules or there are competing rules, and so we have no choice but to choose for ourselves.

This is the case even in health and nursing situations where we're junior and seem to have little autonomy. Whatever our level – novice or expert – we frequently have no option other than to judge personally.

As an initial healthcare example, consider these fairly commonplace circumstances:

SCENARIO 1.1: CULTURALLY COMPETENT?

CATEGORIES: CULTURE, RESPECT

Mrs Suleiman is a 70-year-old widow who's recently had surgery to replace her hip joint, following a fall in which she fractured her neck of femur. She's a patient on your ward.

Mrs Suleiman does not speak English well. She's very family oriented and lives for her children and grandchildren. She loves to cook and can't wait to get fit enough to go home. She's used to having her decisions made by her family, collectively.

Aashif, 30, is Mrs Suleiman's youngest son. He still lives in the family home, though his three brothers and two sisters have now left. Aashif – a devout Muslim – is fiercely protective of his mother.

Aashif is angry that a male physiotherapist and nurse are caring for his mother. He insists that both men must cease treating his mother immediately. He says his mother's wishes must be respected. He will initiate legal action tomorrow if it does not stop.

What should you do for the best? Do you agree with the proposal below?

It is proposed that male health professionals will remain a part of the team caring for Mrs Suleiman.

Now consider a second real-life nursing example:

SCENARIO 1.2: NOVICE VERSUS EXPERT? (CHILD VERSION)

CATEGORIES: DUTY, EMPLOYMENT, NEGLIGENCE

Imagine you're a second year nursing student, based in a community Children's Centre. This is your second placement. You're about to attend a Multidisciplinary Team (**MDT**) meeting to review the multi-professional assessment of one of the children who visit the centre on a daily basis.

On your way to the meeting room you're chatting pleasantly with Katie, a senior worker, who's your assessor for this placement. You're stopped by a small boy named Adam, who's coming the other way along the corridor. He pulls at your trousers vigorously, demanding your attention. You look down and see that he seems very upset. He's stammering, struggling to get his words out, and repeatedly pointing at two other boys who are peering from a door off the corridor.

You cut off your conversation with Katie in mid-sentence to try to talk to Adam, who is now stamping his feet and flapping his arms. Before you can work out his needs, Katie orders him to go to the 'time out' chair in the playroom. She tells him it's very rude to interrupt grown-ups when they're talking, and he needs to sit quietly and think about his behaviour.

You've met Adam briefly on this placement. You know he's 7 years old, attends daily, and is being assessed by a range of professionals, through play and targeted observation. It's currently believed that he may have a form of Autism. He has a significant language development delay and is often disruptive in the playroom – he frequently lashes out at other children, as well as members of staff, when he feels frustrated or unable to communicate his needs. This results in Adam being put in the 'time out' corner of the playroom, which seems to infuriate him further. This intervention is usually initiated by Katie, who regularly explains her reasoning that disruptive children need to be segregated in order to change negative and unsociable behaviour.

Adam starts to cry. Katie tells you – in front of Adam – he's a very difficult child who seems to have no boundaries or respect for others, and that he's an 'attention seeker', and

(Continued)

comes from a 'very rough family'. She says you need to be firmer with him or he will take advantage of your kind nature and have you running around in circles.

Then she stops, with a sigh. 'Look,' she says, 'I know it's not ideal but we just don't have the resources to give everyone individual attention whenever they demand it. They're asking for two voluntary redundancies here, and no-one's opting for that so things are very tense. Edith's putting us all under pressure to increase efficiency, and they reckon her job's not safe either.'

'She's chairing this **MDT** and we don't know why. It's not normal for the boss to do this so we're all a bit worried, to say the least.'

Katie turns to head back along the corridor. She tells you to hurry up and makes it clear she expects you to follow her. Adam's still crying and tugging at your trousers.

You feel troubled and unsure about what's really wrong – and what, if anything, you should do about it.

How do you decide? What should you do? Should you stay and try to help Adam? Or should you obey your assessor and walk away?

Both scenarios are realistic and, therefore, highly complex. You can decide what to do fast or slow – or something in between – but what you definitely cannot do is feed the circumstances into a simple decision-making model, push a button, and churn out the best answer. To decide what to do **you** have to engage personally – as is the case with all the scenarios in this book.

To help reinforce this point, think about a third everyday nursing and healthcare illustration: what to do about a 'difficult' patient. How would this judgement actually be made? And how – if at all – would nursing models and theories help make it?

SCENARIO 1.3: THE WOMAN AND THE DOG

CATEGORIES: LAW, RESOURCES, AUTONOMY

This case concerns a 60-year-old widowed patient with full capacity and no identified mental health problems. She has an extensive and well-documented history of frequent emergency department visits, calling ambulances and coming into the department with her small dog.

When the patient brings her dog into the department she can skip queues – since the dog has to be kept outside for health and safety reasons – and she gets all the attention and care she demands (including hot drinks, food and blankets for her, and a bowl of water for the dog) because she has to wait outside with her pet.

On each occasion the patient complains of acute, severe abdominal pain experienced before arriving at the department; however, this quickly subsides once she's there. No objective evidence of illness can be found when emergency staff assess her, so she's always discharged back home, following examination and various tests.

She's here today. Her dog is barking continuously, annoying and upsetting some of the other patients waiting inside. The emergency department staff, who have to keep popping out to check if she's all right, are becoming increasingly frustrated.

Jessica is the nurse in charge of triage. She's known the woman for over two years and considers her to be a time-waster. She simply doesn't like her. She tries to hide it but worries that she can't. She doesn't want to appear callous but can see no end to the saga.

Her colleague, Simon, a seasoned A&E nurse, walks over to Jessica, three hours after the patient and her dog arrived.

'Don't you think you should see her now? She's been here a long time today.'

Jessica sighs and flushes. 'Why should I?' she says, and slams an NHS rule-book in front of him.

A&E INITIAL ASSESSMENT TRIAGE CATEGORY

1. **Immediate resuscitation.**
2. <u>**PATIENTS**</u> **in need of immediate treatment for preservation of life.**
3. **Very urgent.**
4. **Seriously ill or injured <u>PATIENTS</u> whose lives are not in immediate danger.**
5. **Urgent.**
6. <u>**PATIENTS**</u> **with serious problems, but apparently stable condition.**
7. **Standard.**
8. **Standard A&E cases without immediate danger or distress.**
9. **Non-urgent.**
10. <u>**PATIENTS**</u> **whose conditions are not true accidents or emergencies.**

'She's a 5,' says Jessica. 'She's always a 5.'

There are two ambulance crew at the desk. They start to nod in agreement.

'Come on mate, we bring her in three or four times a month. She gets seen. There's nothing wrong. The bloody dog yaps all the time. Then we take her home again, after a few hours of fun and attention. What about all the other patients we have had to delay getting to?', one says.

'Sally's right,' says the other. 'We need to put a stop to this. Just refuse to see her. Enough's enough.'

Simon becomes agitated, torn between concern for the woman, other patients, the department, and colleagues. He doesn't know what to do but feels – somehow – that the woman should not be rejected.

Just then the patient moves to the desk, dragging her dog with her. The staff look anxious. Has she heard them?

She walks awkwardly up to the desk.

'It's so cold outside and I can't leave him.' She bursts into tears.

(Continued)

Simon is the first to react. He moves over and gently puts his arm around her.

'Come over here. You can sit in my office with your dog until you're seen.'

'How are you feeling at the moment?' he inquires, as he guides her away from the waiting area.

Simon sits her down and says he'll be back with a hot drink soon. He walks, slightly nervously, back to the desk to talk to Jessica and the ambulance team. Another patient, who's been waiting over two hours, has joined them. She's getting progressively more angry.

'Why is that woman getting special treatment? How come she can bring a dog in? I've been bleeding from my leg since I fell – hours ago – and it hasn't stopped. How come she's more important than I am?'

'We have rules and procedures we must stick to,' Jessica responds, desperately hoping to sound convincing.

'Look, I'm badly injured and she isn't so what's that all about?'

As calmly as he can, Simon says, 'We can't always be precise and we're supposed to see everyone who arrives within a certain time, so we can be fair.'

'I've been here hours already and I'm bleeding badly,' the patient protests.

'Please return to your seat and I'll talk to you shortly,' Simon says, firmly.

As the patient obeys, Jessica opens both palms to the ceiling and raises her eyebrows, 'See?'

Simon leans forward so as not to be heard by the patients. 'Yes we see her a lot and we don't know clinically what's wrong. But surely there's something wrong and it's our job to help her if we can. Isn't it?'

What should be done?

(48)

HOW MIGHT NURSING DECISION-MAKING MODELS AND THEORIES HELP DEAL WITH THE WOMAN AND THE DOG?

The simple answer is that nursing models and theories don't help much at all. They may provide a prompt or two, but beyond that much more is required than they can possibly give.

There are no protocols for 'the case of the woman and the dog', no specific laws, and no clear ethical guidance. Presumably any carer would want to support everyone involved and to try not to cause harm, but beyond that it's all a matter of judgement, much of which will be unconscious, 'fast thinking'.

Take the **general decision-making model** described above, for example:

1. Identify the problem
2. Gather evidence
3. List ways to solve the problem
4. Compare and evaluate these
5. Choose the best option
6. Take action accordingly
7. Review the process in case it happens again

The very first step is enough to show the difficulty: 'identify the problem'. Is there actually a problem, and if there is, is it clinical? Social? Is the patient physically ill? Is she mentally ill? Is there a real clinical problem to uncover, or is the patient a hypochondriac? Is the problem the staff? Have they come to dislike the woman unreasonably? Do they have an inappropriate attitude? Is it a problem of education? Are the other patients selfish? Or is this essentially a resource problem? If there were more staff would they be able to cope better? If there were more time to research the woman's claims, would there be a better outcome?

The problem does not identify itself. It's not obvious, and neither is the solution to whatever the problem is judged to be.

The McCloskey and Bulecheck model above (Figure 1.3) refers to patient priorities, involvement and preferences. But in this case these preferences themselves appear to be at least part of the problem. How can they be included in the solution if they're causing the issue in the first place? Most of the healthcare professionals involved disagree with the patient's priorities, so should her preferences be included at all? But if they are not, what priorities should be put in their place? And what does it say about this decision-making model if it's acceptable to dismiss patient preferences whenever they are troublesome?

Clearly, these big questions cannot possibly be resolved by the McCloskey and Bulecheck model on its own. Gibbs' 'reflective cycle' is similarly problematic. To apply Gibbs' model the user must say 'what happened', as a first step. But – apart from the basic, undisputed facts – 'what happened?' or 'what's happening' is a matter of interpretation.

Nursing models and theories merely outline different, largely superficial takes on decision-making. They don't explain how nurses address – or should address – complex human problems in everyday practice. They're more like a silhouette view of different types of car, or a line drawing of cars' shapes, than a manual that explains what they're made of and how they work.

NURSES ARE COMPLEX PEOPLE WHO WORK IN COMPLEX CIRCUMSTANCES

Because nurses are complex people, extensively influenced by many and varied life factors, it's inevitable that different nurses will come to different conclusions when they attempt to solve everyday problems. To those who seek regularity this may seem troubling, unpredictable, uncertain – too messy. But – as we explain in detail in **Chapter Four** – in our view this is exactly as it should be, so long as each decision-maker is willing and able to explain her judgements to herself and others.

Consider a handful of commonplace clinical circumstances:

- Choosing a mattress for a frail elderly man who's been admitted with an acute bowel obstruction.
- Choosing a time to begin asthma education for newly diagnosed patients with asthma.

- Choosing how to approach cardiac rehabilitation with an elderly patient who has had an acute myocardial infarction and lives alone with her family nearby.
- Choosing how to organize handover so that communication is most effective.
- Deciding to use the Edinburgh Postnatal Depression screening tool, rather than anything else.
- Information seeking: the choice to seek (or not seek) further information before making a clinical decision. **(49)**

These, and countless thousands similar, everyday challenges do not have textbook answers. Simple models cannot resolve them on their own. Every nurse must think carefully and combine an array of factors, as she personally sees fit, in order to determine the best course of action, in perpetual uncertainty. Consider: what factors would be most important to you about choosing the mattress for the frail elderly man? Cost? Size? Comfort? Availability? Safety? Hygiene? Durability? If you have to make a compromise – say between cost and safety, or between comfort and durability – how would you decide? Unless one factor is the only one that ever matters, which is obviously not the case, you'll need to use your own judgement. And then, what if the client hates the mattress you prefer? How important is his judgement?

Is there an ideal time to begin asthma education for newly diagnosed sufferers? And is there an ideal form of education? Classes? Individual tuition in a clinical setting? Reading materials? Online learning? Online communities? Peer support? It's far from easy to decide. Different experts advise different methods. There's considerable evidence, yet the more evidence there is the more confusing it becomes to work out what's best **(50)**.

This sentence from the asthma guideline provides a perfect summary:

It cannot be assumed that a successful intervention in one setting will be feasible or appropriate in another.

Working out what's best to do in normal, everyday practice is the central task for nurses. I've read all the evidence, but how should I interpret it? Which authority should I trust? This research paper looks good, but it was funded by a company with an interest in the results turning out well for them. And the results in this other paper are different. My boss says the right answer is obvious, but it doesn't look that way to me. Should I agree to this patient's request today, or should I 'wait and see'? I'm just not sure what's best. Should I use this well-being scale, or a different one – the results come out differently, dependent on which one I use. Which clinical pathway should I use? Which law should I follow? Which statements in the ethical code should I apply in this case? And what do I take each one to mean?

DEFINING PERSONAL JUDGEMENT

The academic literature offers much advice about how to think – from how to analyse decisions with mathematical precision to how to become more 'emotionally intelligent'.

Yet whenever you reflect on how you make decisions as a human being, there's an obvious gap between scholarly treatises and the reality of personal judgement.

Technically, we might define personal judgement very simply, like this:

Personal judgement occurs when a person interprets circumstances.

For example, 'this is good' or 'this is a problem' or 'this is right' or 'this is wrong' or 'this is meaningless' or 'this is relevant' or 'this is irrelevant' or 'we should do this' or 'we should not do this'.

As she makes a personal judgement, a person brings herself (everything that makes her who she is at that point in time) to the circumstances and appraises them from this unique perspective.

This definition has the following implications:

1. Different people can view exactly the same set of circumstances and come to conflicting judgements. For example, two people might see a boy eating a double cheeseburger in a restaurant. One (the restaurant owner) might think 'this is good' while the other (a dietician) might think 'this is a problem'.
2. While circumstances are what they are in the raw, the person judging them is always unique. Therefore, the person and the circumstances combined always create unique situations.
3. The same person can view the same or similar set of circumstances she viewed previously and come to a different judgement, either consciously or unconsciously, if she's changed in some way.

    This is counter-intuitive since we tend to see ourselves as fixed, predictable beings. However, because we're so complex we're much more changeable than we assume. And when we mix ourselves with complicated circumstances, change should not surprise us.

4. Despite repeated references to 'clinical judgement' and 'professional judgement' in the literature, there are no different categories of judgement. Ultimately, all human judgements are personal, they merely occur in different contexts.

SUMMARY OF CHAPTER ONE

1) We don't fully understand how we make decisions
2) We tend to imagine we make our judgements steadily, according to standard processes and pathways
3) In fact, most of our thinking is 'fast' and unconscious
4) Most nursing decision-making models assume 'slow thinking'

(Continued)

5) When the models are applied to real-life circumstances they are of limited use, and may even mislead us

6) A simple definition of personal judgement is that:

Personal judgement occurs when a person interprets circumstances. For example, 'this is good' or 'this is a problem' or 'this is right' or 'this is wrong' or 'this is meaningless' or 'this is relevant' or 'this is irrelevant' or 'we should do this' or 'we should not do this'.

We believe it's infinitely better to accept that generalised rules are never enough – and that often there simply are no rules – rather than pretending that there are authoritative protocols that guarantee 'the correct decisions'.

CHAPTER ONE EXERCISES

Having read **Chapter One** you may like to attempt the following exercises, to reinforce your learning:

1. Reflect on a personal judgement you have made today and attempt to explain why you made it rather than an alternative judgement. What mental and physical processes were involved in your judgement?
2. Take one or more nursing decision-making models and give examples where they can be effectively used for problem-solving
3. Take one or more nursing decision-making models and give examples where they are of little or no use for problem-solving, and explain what is lacking
4. Consider and explain how you, personally, would try to deal with the example of the woman and the dog
5. Describe the personal processes involved as you decided what to do about the woman and the dog. What was happening to you as you decided?

CHAPTER 2

CLASSIC APPROACHES TO NURSING AND HEALTHCARE DECISION-MAKING

AIMS

This chapter has the following aims:

1) To briefly describe and explain ten different, commonly used approaches to nursing decision-making
2) To place these on the **Spectrum**
3) To explain how each can be useful
4) To apply each approach to real-world situations
5) To demonstrate where each approach reaches a point where it is no longer useful
6) To demonstrate that personal judgement is necessary in order to make any decision once this point is reached

LEARNING OUTCOMES

When you have read and worked through this chapter you should be able to:

1) Describe different classic approaches to decision-making
2) Apply these constructively to nursing and healthcare scenarios
3) Identify the points at which personal judgement is needed when applying any of the approaches
4) Offer your own example scenarios from nursing and healthcare and apply your preferred approach(es) to decide what best to do

In this chapter we briefly introduce ten specific ways of deciding what to do in healthcare. These are:

- The Nursing and Midwifery Council (**NMC**) Code of Ethics
- The Law
- Cost–benefit analysis
- Risk avoidance
- Evidence-based practice
- Values-based practice
- The 'four principles'
- Nursing Ethics
- Intuition
- The Ethical Grid

We explain an eleventh – our theory of **PSP** – in **Chapter Four**. It's possible (roughly and very arguably) to place all eleven approaches on nursing's decision-making spectrum, like this:

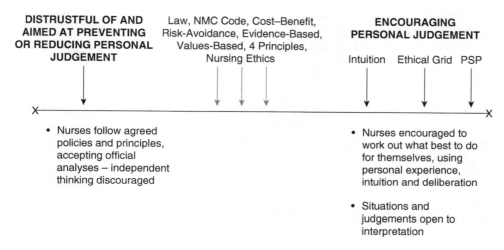

Figure 2.1   Spectrum 2. Some Common Approaches to Decision-Making

Of these methods, eight sit to the left of the spectrum. Each of these eight – one way or another – is suspicious of personal judgement, and seeks to reduce its influence. The other three sit more towards the right, though to what extent is itself a matter of judgement.

The Nursing and Midwifery Council (**NMC**) **Code of Ethics (28)** is a set of general instructions; for example, that you should 'prioritise people' by '... mak[ing] their care and safety your main concern and mak(ing) sure that their dignity is preserved and their needs are recognised, assessed and responded to'.

The **law** is a set of rules created by statutes or the courts that changes over time. It is usually seen as binding on citizens.

Cost–benefit analysis is a process of working out how much good an action will produce, at what price **(51)**.

Risk avoidance is a set of strategies – often laws or parts of Ethical Codes – designed to reduce or eliminate perceived harms **(52)**.

Evidence-based practice (EBP) is based on research results about techniques and their outcomes, and on evidence of patient preferences. If it is clear that a particular technique is likely to bring about the most favourable outcome then it is commonly assumed that everyone should use it **(53)**.

Values-based practice (VBP) is a way to guide behaviours and actions based on shared and agreed values. For example, if it is agreed that 'honesty' is a desirable value then, according to values-based practice, any health carer should be 'honest' in any circumstances **(54)**.

The **'four principles'** are widely cited slogans supposed to be sufficient to guide all health carers to the 'ethical conclusion' in any circumstances. The principles are 'beneficence', 'non-maleficence', 'justice' and 'respect autonomy' **(55)**.

Nursing ethics is based on traditional ethical theory, for example about 'rights', 'duties' and 'principles', applied to the nursing context.

Intuition, it is argued, is a largely unconscious process of pattern recognition that grows and improves with experience.

The **Ethical Grid** is a decision-making tool used in some courses on healthcare ethics. It consists of 20 tiles that display key concepts such as 'create autonomy', 'truth' and 'resources available', which a decision-maker can define and choose as she sees fit, in order to make and justify decisions **(20)**.

We will consider these approaches in more detail below. But first it's important to expand on certain complexities briefly outlined earlier, since making decisions, even with the help of these methods, is more complicated, challenging and more mysterious than it may seem.

TWO FURTHER COMMONPLACE HEALTHCARE SCENARIOS

In order to explore these complexities, consider two further everyday healthcare scenarios – one concerning truth-telling, the other to do with forcibly restraining a patient. Since these are not unusual challenges, one might expect there to be generally agreed answers about what to do for the best. But – as we are learning – healthcare practice is not like this.

As you reflect on the examples, try to observe the process that occurs within you, as a human being, as you attempt to make the right judgement. Try to notice what you bring with you as you decide. Try to notice how you are personally affected and how that in turn affects the way you see the situation.

What happens to **you** as **you** decide what to do?

——— SCENARIO 2.1: WHERE'S MY WIFE? ———

CATEGORIES: DEMENTIA, CANDOUR, SAFEGUARDING, RESPECT

Joe, 78, lives alone in a specially adapted bungalow. He is supported by a comprehensive community care package, provided by Social Services.

Joe suffers from Vascular Dementia and Chronic Obstructive Pulmonary Disease (**COPD**). Four years ago he suffered a Cerebral Vascular Accident (**CVA**), which caused some mild residual perception effect, arising from the occipital region of his brain, causing Joe to be clumsy and more likely to bump into things and people in his peripheral vision. The **CVA** occurred after it was discovered that he was suffering from hypertension and high cholesterol. However, both conditions are now well managed with medication.

Joe's wife, Alice, passed away three years ago. Joe was diagnosed with dementia after he was found wandering and lost by the police two years ago. At this point Joe and his daughter both decided it would be best for Joe to stay in his own home as long as possible, to avoid further confusion and disorientation. Joe enjoys being at home, with his personal belongings and photos of his wife around him. It appears this helps Joe to stay oriented to time and place.

Joe has been relatively stable for the last year. Currently he appears to have fluctuating capacity to make decisions, dependent on context and time of day. Joe is fairly lucid during the mornings but tends to become more confused at night time, especially if he needs to get out of bed to use the bathroom. Joe has a sleep-in carer who supports his needs at night.

At the moment Joe is fully mobile. He's not incontinent of urine and has no muscle weakness or seizures. However, this is expected to change as the course of his illness progresses.

Joe is visited by the Dementia Specialist Nurse on a monthly basis. He also has a daughter who calls on him once a day in the late morning, to prepare meals for him to heat up in his microwave.

You are a community health professional visiting Joe, in the late afternoon, in order to assess his current needs and management of his **COPD**. Joe is currently suffering from a mild chest infection, which seems to have brought about more confusion than normal. Joe's been forgetting when mealtimes are and when to take his routine and daily medications, which is rarely a problem normally.

Following a visit by the duty GP, Joe is now being treated with appropriate antibiotics and has been improving over the last few days, however he's still somewhat more confused than normal, according to the sleep-in carer and his daughter.

While visiting and assessing Joe, he suddenly asks you where his wife is. At this moment you are unsure how to respond to him.

What would you do in this situation?

It is proposed that you tell a white lie – such as 'she is at the shops'.

Do you agree?

How would you feel if put on the spot like this? How would you feel emotionally? How would you feel physically? Try to think about your heart rate, your breathing. Are you blushing? Are you anxious? Calm? Assertive? Assured? Uncertain? Panicked? How logical would you feel?

SCENARIO 2.2: ELAINE

CATEGORIES: LEARNING DISABILITIES, SAFEGUARDING, RESPECT, CONSENT

Elaine is a 27-year-old woman who has a severe learning disability. She's currently detained under the Mental Health Act.

Elaine finds it difficult to tolerate any requests and demands placed on her. She finds any close contact from carers or other residents impossible to cope with. If she feels threatened she will barge at people with enough force to knock them off their feet.

(Continued)

All personal care, washing, dressing, oral hygiene and so on has to be done with great care to avoid distress. This often means that only the very basic hygiene is achieved.

A major concern is the condition of her hair, which is heavily matted and tangled and has been described as resembling 'upright dreadlocks'. Elaine does not seem bothered by her hair's condition. She often puts spittle on her hands and then strokes them through her hair, adding to the hair hygiene problem.

Staff report that Elaine will allow water to be put on her hair and that they attempt to use a 'de-frizz' shampoo but she won't allow them to massage this in. Staff have tried to use conditioner to soften the hair and allow easier brushing or combing but Elaine will not endure this. They have also used mild sedation and short duration physical intervention, but this caused Elaine too much distress for them to continue.

Elaine's mother, who still has close contact with her daughter, has asked that her daughter's hair be cut. She says Elaine used to have 'nice hair' and used to enjoy how it made her look.

Staff are also concerned that there are possible health risks because of the condition of Elaine's hair – head lice, psoriasis and alopecia, though none of these conditions currently exist.

Do you cut Elaine's hair?

It is proposed that Elaine is restrained and her hair is cut.

Do you agree? How would you feel if you had to decide what best to do for Elaine?

HOW DO YOU DECIDE WHICH APPROACH TO USE TO DECIDE WHAT TO DO?

These two scenarios are difficult enough as it is. However, there's a further level of difficulty beyond the decisions themselves.

If the decision-makers are to be consistent – and as we have seen it is widely recommended in nursing and healthcare that they should be – they should presumably use the same approach. However, there are no rules in 'no right answer' cases to indicate which (or which combination) of the 11 approaches should be used. So, somehow, not only must the health carers work out what to decide in the absence of objective rules, but they must also work out which method to choose to help them decide in the absence of definitive guidance.

Let's pause to take stock, since this phenomenon is repeatedly skated over in the literature. We've seen that consistency and uniformity is often held to be preferable to autonomous judgement in nursing, and yet in everyday circumstances where there are no simple rules to follow, standardised guidance is not possible. Even if health carers X and Y both happen to choose the same approach to a problem, to be consistent they must both define it and apply it in the same way. But sooner or later it's inevitable that different health carers will choose different approaches and therefore make different decisions.

In short, personal judgement is required to:

1. Identify a problem. (Is this a problem? To whom is it a problem? Does everyone involved agree there's a problem? Does everyone see it the same way?)
2. To decide the best approach to use to try to solve the problem.
3. To define the details of the approach – for example, to state which part of a professional Code or law of the land to use, or to calculate how to weigh the cost of a particular option, or to decide which ethical value is most appropriate.
4. To apply the approach to the particular problem (how do I use this risk analysis in these circumstances?).
5. To decide which solution is most acceptable to others involved.
6. To decide which solution is most acceptable to oneself.
7. To offer a justification of your chosen solution.

Let's consider Joe and Elaine a little more.

NO ABSOLUTE RULES

There are no absolute rules that can help decide what to do for either Joe or Elaine. Walking away is not a neutral option either. That would be a choice not to tell Joe and choice to accept the status quo in Elaine's case.

If you're an advocate of any of the approaches we describe in this chapter – if you usually resort to ethical codes or the law or cost-benefit analysis, for example – then you may be struggling to work out how to apply your approach to decide what to do for Joe and Elaine.

As we have already noted, most ethical codes tell practitioners that they must 'act in the best interests' of patients or clients:

4. Act in the best interests of people at all times

To achieve this, you must:

4.1 balance the need to act in the best interests of people at all times with the requirement to respect a person's right to accept or refuse treatment

4.2 make sure that you get properly informed consent and document it before carrying out any action.

The **NMC** Code also advises, in ten different places, not to cause avoidable harm:

You must:

17.1 take all reasonable steps to protect people who are vulnerable or at risk from harm, neglect or abuse. **(28)**

But the Code is unable to explain, even in general, never mind in Joe's and Elaine's particular cases, how to balance 'acting in best interests' with respecting the person's rights.

Nor can it tell the decision-maker how to protect Joe and Elaine from harm, since it's not even clear what 'harm' means in either case.

The law can't help much either. It can tell you what not to do – deliberately cause harm to either patient, for example – but it can't tell you what positive intervention to offer. Both telling the truth and avoiding it in Joe's case, and cutting her hair or not in Elaine's case, are legal options.

Cost–benefit analysis has the same limitations. You need to know exactly what costs and benefits are involved in order to calculate an acceptable ratio between them – ideally maximising benefits and minimising costs. But at the moment this is unknowable. Telling Joe the truth, or not telling him, could be either a cost or a benefit, dependent upon what happens, and on how you judge it. And it is the same for Elaine's haircut.

However detailed and complex each approach is – and they can be very complex – we believe that personal judgement is much more important. Not only is it absolutely necessary to use personal judgement to decide what approaches to use, but judgement is also required to specify what each approach actually means in practice, whenever you want to change any situation.

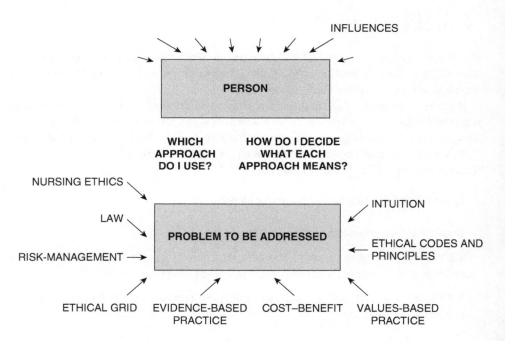

Figure 2.2   Personal Judgement is Required to Choose and Define Approaches to Decision-Making

WHAT TO DO FOR JOE?

We know – from actual debates about these issues on the Values Exchange (**56**) over nearly two decades – that some people (including those with years of experience in dementia care) will choose to tell Joe the truth and others will either lie or delay telling him.

There are no objective justifications. There is no oracle of truth – just different personal judgements about the circumstances we encounter.

We will consider the options for Joe in more detail in **Chapter Four**.

WHAT TO DO FOR ELAINE?

Like most scenarios in this book, Elaine's case is based on real events. It caused considerable distress to Learning Disabilities staff working in a UK NHS Trust, who simply could not decide what best to do. Some were in favour of cutting Elaine's hair, others were opposed, others said they would go along with the majority, and most wavered from time to time. The dilemma persisted for several months and was debated extensively in staff meetings and also on an early version of the Values Exchange, on which everyone could have a say – anonymously or not – without pressure or fear of recrimination.

Different staff put forward different reasons for and against a haircut. What was most striking was that it became obvious to everyone that there was no objective viewpoint. There was no official authority – no rule-book – that could be used to arbitrate. Everyone could see that the issue needed to be resolved through caring conversation, between all the human beings involved.

What helped the most was the opportunity for staff and relatives to talk, to try to reach a decision together: to be heard and to be respected. The opportunity to debate safely, and to consider all points of view defused all previous conflicts. Everyone could see that everyone else's point of view was included.

In the end, everyone agreed that whether Elaine's hair was cut or not mattered less and less. All involved concluded that, because of the sensitive discussion process, they could accept both cutting or not cutting. Everyone had been respected as an individual person, and no one had tried to impose an artificial, arbitrary set of rules.

In the end it was agreed not to cut Elaine's hair, unless its condition became a clear threat to the health and well-being of other clients, at which point it would be cut as gently as possible with calming music and scents.

It is, however, quite pointless and misleading to say that this was 'the right answer'.

THE APPROACHES

It's possible to apply any of the approaches to try to arrive at a decision about any of the scenarios we present in this book. Whatever approach is used, sooner or later (and usually sooner) there comes a point where something more is required. There are few exceptions to this rule. Unless the decision is technical and closed – for example, deciding which of only two possible medications is best to use, or deciding which vein is easiest to take blood from – the decision-maker has to make a choice beyond the scope of the approach she has chosen to apply.

To understand a little more detail, let's take the approaches and apply them to another healthcare example – there are endless examples after all.

—— SCENARIO 2.3: DYING FOR A DRAG? ——

CATEGORIES: TERMINAL ILLNESS, PATIENT CHOICE, RIGHTS, DUTY

You are a health worker on a medium dependency surgical ward.

Tom is a 56-year-old patient with terminal lung cancer and bony metastases. Tom currently lives alone. Although he's normally independent and mobile, he appears profoundly fatigued, fragile and thin. He's on continuous oxygen therapy, via nasal cannulae, and has been admitted to the ward for post-operative care and rehabilitation.

Tom fell at home recently, suffering a pathological fracture to his right shaft of femur. Yesterday he had an open reduction and internal fixation during surgery.

Tom is expected to be discharged from the ward in about three to four days, following physiotherapy, occupational therapy and health and social care assessments. He's expected to stay with his brother James, following discharge. Tom reluctantly agreed to this following a concerted discussion, initiated by James, who plans to care for Tom until he regains most of his previous mobility, at which point Tom says he will return home alone, which is his strong preference since he is very protective of the autonomy he still has.

Tom has remained a 40-a-day smoker since he was diagnosed 18 months ago, despite pressure to stop from his doctors and family. He says he enjoys smoking too much – it's one of the only things he continues to find pleasurable in his life as it is now. Tom's siblings describe Tom as 'stubborn' and 'someone who doesn't take orders from others'. They also suggest that as soon as Tom is able to mobilise, he'll most probably find a way to go outside, or to a toilet to smoke a cigarette.

You are assigned to care for Tom on the late shift. During the evening, Tom's siblings visit and enter his private room. You clearly witness them hand an electronic vapour cigarette to Tom. You're surprised by this and also concerned because – since recent EU directives have come into force – the hospital has both a smoking and e-cigarette ban that operates across all its buildings and grounds.

You offer to ask the doctor to prescribe nicotine replacement patches for Tom but Tom says he finds these ineffective and prefers an e-cigarette, as it feels more like a real cigarette. You offer other alternatives such as gum but at this point Tom becomes anxious, agitated and cross, which visibly increases his respiratory effort.

What would you do in this situation? Do you agree or disagree with the proposal?

It is proposed that you take Tom's e-cigarette away from him.

How might each approach help, and how might the choice of approach affect the outcome?

THE LAW

Let's take the law first. Let's say, for example, that you think this must be a legal issue, and that therefore you do not have to make a personal judgement, rather you need merely abide by the law. After all, there's a comprehensive ban on smoking in place in the hospital, you're employed by the hospital, your job is to follow hospital policy and to apply the law, preventing Tom from smoking his e-cigarette must be the only option: case closed, no further judgement required.

But of course the law does not eliminate the need for personal judgement. In fact you've already used it. You did so in the first place, when you decided to use the law to solve your problem. This decision did not make itself. You didn't have to choose the law; you could have used any of the other approaches instead, on their own or in some combination. You might, for instance, have decided that Tom's case is an ethical issue rather than a legal one. Or you might have resolved to undertake a risk or cost–benefit calculation. It was up to you, the existence of a law does not oblige you to follow it.

LEGAL AND UNETHICAL — ETHICAL AND ILLEGAL

We are aware that this conclusion may surprise some readers, so it's perhaps worth a little further clarification. We are not saying that health professionals should randomly break the law. However, we are saying that:

1. there may be circumstances where other outcomes are more important (for example, breaking the speed limit in order to get to A&E to save a person's life)
2. there are times where you can choose one law over another, and that this is a matter of judgement (for example, you may find respecting a person's privacy more important than keeping them as safe as possible, or you may decide to use the law of tort rather than the duty of candour since these are not always compatible – telling a person a painful truth they did not want to hear and harming them as a result could be regarded as negligent, so it is up to you to choose which law to use)
3. there are 'bad laws' that people can and do choose to break to bring about what they see as better consequences (for example, health professionals striking to bring about better patient care; breaking racial segregation laws in the interests of equality; civil disobedience – refusal to obey laws as a way of forcing a government to do or change something such as furthering workers' or gender rights).

Just because a law exists, this does not necessarily make it reasonable to use it. Laws exist as a matter of fact, but it is up to each of us to decide to obey or apply them. Not only that, but laws come and go. So merely saying 'I must do this because it's the law' is simply not an objective judgement.

In the past there have been societies with no specific laws, and there are currently societies with very different laws from each other. For example, some countries permit abortion and others do not, so it is not possible to look to the law for a definitive ethical judgement even about life and death matters.

In medieval times it was legal to hunt witches, to 'hang, draw and quarter' people who had committed petty theft and to capture and sell slaves. Most people today would not consider such practices ethical, or even particularly sane. And it is the same in the present – laws that exist now will be overturned and new laws that do not presently exist will be passed. Practices that are now thought to be legal and ethical will become illegal and unethical and *vice versa*. Possible examples include: the sale and possession of guns; the manufacture of cars capable of exceeding speed limits; assisted suicide; compulsory schooling of children; punishment for parents who choose to take their children on vacation during term time; stealing from supermarkets to feed a starving child; the ability of companies to report people to credit agencies if they are a little late paying bills; the docking of sheep and cow tails by farmers without anaesthetic; and the mistreatment of animals while in transit to slaughterhouses or while they are being farmed, or indeed the farming of livestock at all. There are very many examples that show that personal judgement about what is right and wrong is immeasurably more important than the law **(20)**.

CURRENT LEGAL JUDGEMENTS

In Tom's case, the next question you need to decide, once you've decided that using the law is the best approach, is 'which law should I follow?'. There's a range of laws to choose from, and the question of which to use does not answer itself automatically.

Furthermore, whether or not a blanket ban on smoking tobacco is lawful or not has been the subject of legal debate and challenge since it was widely introduced in 2011. Currently (2019), it appears to be partially lawful in the case of tobacco at least **(57)**. But this may not remain the case, seems not to apply to e-cigarettes, and it certainly does not apply to the **possession** of smoking materials, including tobacco.

In brief, the story is as follows:

Two patients detained at low and medium secure psychiatric units in Scotland claimed that the blanket ban on smoking in the grounds of the mental health hospitals, which had been enforced since 2105, extending the 2011 prohibition of smoking indoors – breached their human rights. This claim was rejected by the UK Supreme Court.

Counsel for the hospitals referred to the duty imposed on the Scottish Ministers by section 1 of the National Health Service (Scotland) Act 1978 to promote in Scotland a comprehensive and integrated health service designed to secure (a) improvement in the physical and mental health of the people of Scotland, and (b) the prevention, diagnosis and treatment of illness, and for that purpose to secure the effective provision of services in accordance with the provisions of the Act.

Section 2A(1) imposed directly a duty on each health board to promote the improvement of the physical and mental health of the people of Scotland, while section 2A(2) provided that a health board may do anything which they consider is likely to assist in discharging that duty.

Using a narrow and contestable definition of 'health', the judge accepted that the protection of the health of patients and staff was a 'legitimate aim' and that there was a 'rational connection' between the ban and that objective. (**57**)

It is, of course, highly arguable whether preventing patients who enjoy smoking from doing so is good for their mental health, but this is the current legal position. Consequently, as a nurse, you could certainly try to use this law to tell Tom not to smoke. However, actually enforcing this rule against Tom's will would be another matter altogether.

First of all, while the court held that the comprehensive ban did not of itself breach the appellant's rights under Article 8 of the European Convention on Human Rights, or under Article 8 read with Article 14, a prohibition on patients' **possession** of tobacco products, with associated confiscations and searches (including 'sources of ignition' like matches and lighters) was found to be unlawful because those matters fell within the scope of the Mental Health (Care and Treatment) (Scotland) Act 2003 and the Mental Health (Safety and Security) (Scotland) Regulations 2005.

In short, at present, patients are not allowed to smoke tobacco in UK hospitals or grounds, but they are allowed to possess both it and the means to smoke it.

THE LAW ON SMOKING TOBACCO DOES NOT EXTEND TO E-CIGARETTES

It's also very unlikely, from the court's ruling, that the law extends to e-cigarettes, which Public Health England (**PHE**) has concluded are '95% safer' than tobacco cigarettes (**58**).

PHE said every smoker struggling to quit, including pregnant women, should be encouraged to take up e-cigarettes and be allowed to vape indoors, even in bed. Officials have encouraged hospitals to replace smoking shelters with vaping lounges. And they said the devices should be given out by GPs on prescription, to encourage wider take-up.

There is an authoritative review of the evidence (as of March 2018) here (**59**).

Overall, the **PHE** has concluded:

e-cigarettes and tobacco cigarettes are not the same and shouldn't be treated as such. It's important that England's seven million smokers are aware of the differences and have accurate information to inform their health decisions. E-cigarettes aren't completely risk free but carry a fraction of the risk of smoking and are helping thousands of smokers to quit and stay smokefree. (**60**)

Some UK hospitals do now allow the smoking of e-cigarettes, at least in hospital grounds (**61**), while still banning tobacco cigarettes (**62**).

According to ITV news:

Dr Stephen Fowlie, medical director at one NHS Trust that permits e-cigarettes, said:

'We have a duty to help our patients and staff make healthy life choices, and can't ignore the potential benefits of electronic cigarettes as a nicotine replacement therapy.

'We're now allowing e-cigarettes on our grounds to give our patients, staff and visitors more choice in how they quit smoking.'

And Professor John Britton, director of the UK Centre for Tobacco & Alcohol Studies and respiratory consultant at the Trust added:

We need to encourage all patients and visitors who smoke and find it difficult to abstain while in hospital grounds to use medicinal nicotine, or an electronic cigarette.

Approving the use of electronic cigarettes is an important step towards achieving completely smoke free hospitals in Nottingham. (**61**)

DISCRIMINATION

What this seems to mean for Tom is that while it may be hospital policy not to allow him to smoke his e-cigarette, this policy is not supported by law. Not to permit Tom to vape as he wishes is, in the absence of a definitive ruling to the opposite, contrary to Article 8 of the **ECHR** and also sections 15 and 19 of the UK *Equality Act* (2010). Legally, preventing Tom from smoking his e-cigarette is likely, in law, to be regarded as discrimination.

Tom is unable to leave the hospital grounds because of his current disabilities. The Equality Act states, Section 15:

Discrimination arising from disability

A person (A) discriminates against a disabled person (B) if:

A treats B unfavourably because of something arising in consequence of B's disability, and A cannot show that the treatment is a proportionate means of achieving a legitimate aim. (**63**)

The idea that you can simply apply 'the law' and so avoid or minimise personal judgement in Tom's case is starting to look highly implausible. Do you allow Tom to smoke his e-cigarette, so risking action against you by your employer if your employer bans vaping? Or do you prevent Tom smoking in order to uphold your employer's rule? Your employment contract is likely to stipulate that you enforce the hospital's policies and rules, and yet legally this is in contravention of Tom's human rights.

You find yourself in a conundrum: damned if you do and damned if you don't.

WHAT IF TOM DECIDES TO VAPE REGARDLESS?

Things get even more complicated if Tom decides to smoke his e-cigarette anyway, despite the official ban.

It is definitely legal for Tom to possess his e-cigarette. If you take it from him without his permission this is simple theft, and you would place yourself at risk of criminal prosecution. Furthermore, if Tom is actually vaping and you physically force him to stop, perhaps by holding his arm or wrestling the e-cigarette from him, then, in law, you have assaulted Tom. Again, you would place yourself at risk of criminal prosecution.

You need to decide what to do. Knowledge of the law can help, up to a point; however, you can choose to use the law to try to justify **both** options – allowing him to smoke (Equality Acts, no specific legislation preventing e-cigarettes, human rights, Trusts not having any legal authority to ban smoking in its grounds) (**64**):

> A hospital trust has started a campaign to discourage visitors from smoking at hospital entrances – because they have no legal power to stop people from lighting up … The hospital, which is run by South Tees Hospitals NHS Foundation Trust, operates a strict no-smoking policy in all buildings and grounds.
>
> But the trust has no way to legally enforce the policy – meaning that smokers regularly smoke close to department entrances.
>
> 'We've done a lot of work to provide stop smoking support to people and to try and prevent smoking in our hospital grounds, the key issue for us is, legally, we cannot enforce a ban on site outside of the hospital buildings,' a spokeswoman said.
>
> 'We can, and rigidly do, impose a smoking ban inside the buildings but we cannot enforce a ban when the smoker is in the open air – even though they are on NHS property.'

And preventing him from smoking (possibly the UK Supreme Court ruling, right of property owners to decide what is permissible in their property (**65**)).

Which course of action you take, what risks you accept, what law you use to justify what you do, and whether you try make justifications for your actions beyond the law, is ultimately up to you. It's a matter of personal judgement.

THE NMC CODE

But perhaps law is simply the wrong approach to choose in Tom's case. Perhaps a better way would be to apply the **NMC's** ethical code (**28**). Tom wants to smoke his e-cigarette, the hospital says he can't. What's the ethical thing to do, according to the **NMC** Code?

Item 1 of the Code says that the nurse should treat people as individuals and uphold their dignity, and that:

> To achieve this, you must:
>
> 1.1 treat people with kindness, respect and compassion …
>
> 1.3 avoid making assumptions and recognise diversity and individual choice …
>
> 1.5 respect and uphold people's human rights

Item 2 says nurses must:

> Listen to people and respond to their preferences and concerns

And:

> 2.1 work in partnership with people to make sure you deliver care effectively.

Item 3 instructs nurses to:

> Make sure that people's physical, social and psychological needs are assessed and responded to and
>
> 3.4 act as an advocate for the vulnerable, challenging poor practice and discriminatory attitudes and behaviour relating to their care.

Item 4 says that nurses should:

> 4. Act in the best interests of people at all times.

The Code also says that nurses should:

> 8.5 work with colleagues to preserve the safety of those receiving care
>
> 8.6 share information to identify and reduce risk …
>
> 19.4 take all reasonable personal precautions necessary to avoid any potential health risks to colleagues, people receiving care and the public …
>
> 20.4 keep to the laws of the country in which you are practising …
>
> 25 Provide leadership to make sure people's wellbeing is protected and to improve their experiences of the healthcare system …
>
> 25.1 identify priorities, manage time, staff and resources effectively and deal with risk to make sure that the quality of care or service you deliver is maintained and improved, putting the needs of those receiving care or services first …

So, while the **NMC Code** is well written and reasonable, it's not specific, and is open to very wide interpretation. Once again, in order to use the Code in any meaningful way in real life, nurses obviously must use their personal judgement.

In Tom's case, just as we found when considering the law, it's clearly possible to use the Code to justify **both** allowing and preventing him from smoking his e-cigarette. The Code says that nurses must act in the 'best interests' of patients at all times, but does not and cannot define what 'best interest' means in specific circumstances. If Tom and his family say it's in Tom's best interest for him to smoke while official policy says it isn't, then the Code offers no realistic resolution of the disagreement.

It's easy to take statements from the Code and say they justify whatever you want them to. For example, if you want to support Tom in his smoking you might use:

> 1.3 avoid making assumptions and recognise diversity and individual choice
>
> 1.5 respect and uphold people's human rights

2. Listen to people and respond to their preferences and concerns

2.1 work in partnership with people to make sure you deliver care effectively

3. Make sure that people's physical, social and psychological needs are assessed and responded to

and

3.4 act as an advocate for the vulnerable, challenging poor practice and discrimina-tory attitudes and behaviour relating to their care.

On the other hand. if you want to prevent Tom smoking you might use:

4. Act in the best interests of people at all times

8.5 work with colleagues to preserve the safety of those receiving care

8.6 share information to identify and reduce risk

19.4 take all reasonable personal precautions necessary to avoid any potential health risks to colleagues, people receiving care and the public ...

You might argue that it's not in Tom's best interest to smoke at all, given his illness. And you might point to the 'health risks' to others of promoting any smoking habit (**66**):

> [e-cigarettes] ... are often marketed as being relatively safe. However, alternative tobacco products contain potentially harmful chemicals and toxins. These may cause serious health problems, including cancer. Because of these risks, the US Food and Drug Administration (FDA) started regulating these products in 2016.

But in the end it is up to you. While thoroughly well-intentioned and caring, the only real service the Code offers to nurses is first to frame nursing as a respectful, compassionate profession, in very general terms, and second to show beyond all doubt the extent and importance of personal judgement in healthcare.

COST–BENEFIT ANALYSIS

Cost–benefit analysis can be a highly technical matter (**67, 68**) and it is, therefore, neither necessary nor helpful to explain this approach in detail in this book. The key point to make – as with all the approaches we outline in this chapter – is that however technical the approach chosen personal judgement is always necessary, and at many levels.

In every instance when a cost–benefit analysis is under consideration, there are at least these choices to make:

1. Should I use cost–benefit analysis or not?
2. Should I use cost–benefit analysis on its own or with other approaches?
3. What do I define as a 'cost'?

4. What do I define as a 'benefit'?
5. How should I contain or 'ring-fence' the analysis? For example, which costs and which benefits do I include and which do I exclude? How far into the future do I include the costs and benefits?
6. Do I ask others (Tom, for example) if they see the same costs and benefits as I do, or do I use only my own opinions?
7. Do I compare my analysis with other options (for example, campaigning to allow e-cigarettes in hospitals) or do I focus only on the most simple circumstances?

All these are matters of judgement. They are not objective choices.

In Tom's case, looking at the seven questions above, it's not clear that a cost–benefit approach is the best choice. This method is probably better suited to more readily quantifiable matters, like assessing financial investments, devising new business strategies, choosing a new job or deciding whether to buy a new house or stay in your present home. But even in these cases, there are still personal judgements to be made. For example, should I develop a mixed portfolio of investments or should I go for the biggest return? Or should I go for the most certain return even if it will not maximise my income?

When considering a house move, which costs and which benefits matters most? How can I even be sure which is a cost and which is a benefit? For example, do I include resale value? Affordability? Location? State of repair? My potential happiness in this home? My partner's potential happiness? My children's?

What are the costs and benefits in Tom's case? Is protecting hospital policy a cost or a benefit? Is promoting Tom's 'health' a cost or a benefit? Who defines these concepts in this case, Tom or I?

Do I consider only the immediate effects of whatever decision I make, or do I look more broadly and longer term?

Even using a mathematical analysis – which cost–benefit typically is – the questions seem endless.

RISK ASSESSMENT

(Adapted from *Thoughtful Health Care*, **69**)

Risks are generally regarded as isolated elements in life, like banana skins on pavements – hazards to be swept up before someone gets hurt. Or they seem like meteors coming at us out of the sky: huge, separate extra-terrestrial boulders to be shot down and destroyed, like aliens in a video game.

But there's a strange phenomenon – the more we try to eradicate risk the more risks there seem to be. It's like the toddlers' toy with plastic clowns hiding in holes on a game board. Whenever a clown pops up the child is supposed to hit him back down with a hammer, yet this merely causes another clown to pop out from another hole, endlessly.

The problem is seeing risks as separate when it makes no sense to do so.

THE STRANGE CASE OF THE DANGEROUS FLOWERS

The UK newspaper, the *Daily Mail*, recently highlighted a bizarre but far from unusual 'healthcare risk', leading with the headline:

FLOWERS BAN AT 9 IN 10 HOSPITALS: INCREASING NUMBERS INTRODUCE RULES AFTER CONCERNS BLOOMS SPREAD GERMS AND CREATE EXTRA WORK FOR NURSES

A splash of colour in an otherwise dreary hospital ward can brighten up even the most difficult of days.

But according to a survey, nine out of ten NHS hospitals do not allow patients to have fresh flowers by their bed – despite three out of four people opposing a ban.

Increasing numbers of hospitals have introduced the rules to address concerns about spreading germs, aggravating allergies and creating extra work for nurses.

However the poll of 3,700 Britons discovered that around 90 per cent said flowers can dramatically improve someone's mood when they are unwell, and almost half thought they would speed up recovery. Just over three-quarters of people surveyed disagreed with banning the gifts.

There's no official ruling from the Department of Health on whether flowers should be allowed in wards. (**70**)

Craft supplier Country Baskets, who conducted the poll said 'we appreciate the concerns around taking flowers on to wards. But there are real, proven benefits to giving flowers to people who are unwell.'

And psychologist Emma Kenny pointed to evidence that 'many studies ... show the psychological impact that flowers can have on a person's recovery or general well-being ...'

Nevertheless, despite the many positives associated with flowers, according to the poll of 105 hospitals there was a fresh flower ban in 97 of them, with the rest discouraging visitors from bringing bouquets.

Apart from the fact that there's no clear evidence of any risk caused by having flowers on wards, there's a much deeper consideration here. Someone or other – maybe a few people, it's unlikely to be more – looked at flowers in hospitals and identified them as 'a risk' – with the emphasis on 'a'. According to these 'risk detectives', flowers on wards are a self-contained problem, which, once prevented, will remove a single risk. Get rid of the flowers – another risk bites the dust. End of story.

But like any other perceived problem, not only is it we who say whether and to what extent something is a risk, but if you get rid of one risk you never do so without consequences. The world is not made up of disconnected elements – it's a rich and deeply interrelated tapestry where affecting one thread is bound to affect other threads, just like the butterfly effect (**71**).

Because we live in a connected world, if you ban flowers you may stop one perceived risk but you're bound to create new ones. Banning 'dangerous flowers', for example, will at the very least cause:

- A less beautiful environment: a ward full of flowers is much prettier than one without them.
- Less happy patients, especially those who love flowers and gardens.
- Reduced psychological well-being and longer recovery times.
- Reduced patient choice and autonomy: if I'm prevented from having flowers at my bedside I am likely to feel disempowered and trapped.
- Conflict between staff and patients/visitors who want to bring in flowers: if I'm visiting my friend in hospital with a bouquet of flowers and I'm prevented from delivering them, not only will I feel frustrated and sad, but I might well end up arguing with the staff member who has to implement the ban, whether it's her choice or not.
- An environment in which the whole notion of risk is inflated beyond what can possibly be considered sensible.
- An environment where patients become increasingly scared and fearful about all the risks they hear about.
- Unnecessary anxiety amongst patients and relatives about having flowers at home when they're sick.
- Demotivation amongst staff who have not been involved in this decision (obviously not everyone agrees with the flower ban, which is an imposed decision – and imposing decisions on people itself brings many risks).
- A ripple effect – or slippery slope – where further quite normal and safe situations and practices fall under the official gaze, as the 'risk bar' is subtly lowered further and further (allowing patients to have books for example could be seen as an infection risk, or possibly an injury hazard, if they are large and heavy books).

Part of the risk phobia problem is lack of institutional imagination, and lack of power – or guts – in employees afraid of the consequences to them as individuals. As soon as someone identifies a perceived risk everyone panics. For example:

'We have to take this seriously. What if it actually happens and we didn't do anything about it?'

'Something has to be done. We have to manage this situation. We can't keep the lid on this. Let's make it official so everyone can see we are managing risk effectively.'

Preventing one risk sets off a cascade of further risks, but this is rarely understood. As a cure I suggest the simplest of questions. Whenever it occurs to someone to prevent a risk they should ask:

What's the risk of preventing this risk?

There will always be further risks. It's just the way things are.
As Allen Buchanan writes:

> Eliminating risk isn't possible. Life isn't like that. But even if it were possible, eliminating risk would be a mistake, because the costs of doing this would be too high …

> Here's an example. Suppose we can achieve a 10% reduction of serious injury in a car crash for every additional one eighth inch of steel we add to the body of a car. If we add enough to make the doors as thick as the hull of an Abrams tank, nobody will die in a car crash …. But beyond a certain point, an additional increment of risk reduction … isn't worth it. The car becomes unaffordable and the cost of gas for such a heavy vehicle becomes prohibitive. (p. 87) **(72)**

As in the children's game, a clown pops up from the hole. Someone hits him. Immediately, a new clown – sometimes several new clowns – pop out of other holes.

Tom's case illustrates the problem well. The initial perceived danger is the risk of the e-cigarette to Tom's health. One solution is to take it away from him. This, of course, creates further risks, in this case the risks of upsetting Tom, causing him to feel a loss of control (having control is a key part of many theories of health), making him less 'compliant', causing him to vape anyway (which in turn creates further risks), causing him to vape in the toilets, or even frustrating him so much that he lights up a real cigarette.

EVIDENCE-BASED DECISION-MAKING

On the face of it, this is a very obvious approach. If you want to make an effective decision then you should assess the evidence and act accordingly. It would seem most strange to advise otherwise. However, as always, on closer inspection things are less straightforward, and personal judgement is required in all but the most routine circumstances.

Generally speaking, evidence-based decision-making (more commonly referred to as evidence-based practice or **EBP**) is based on three key factors:

> Evidence-based practice is a conscientious, problem-solving approach to clinical practice that incorporates the best evidence from well-designed studies, patient values and preferences, and a clinician's expertise in making decisions about a patient's care. Unfortunately, no standard formula exists for how much these factors should be weighed in the clinical decision-making process. However, there are a variety of rating systems and hierarchies of evidence that grade the strength or quality of evidence generated from a research study or report. Being knowledgeable about evidence-based practice and levels of evidence is important to every clinician as clinicians need to be confident about how much emphasis they should place on a study, report, practice alert or clinical practice guideline when making decisions about a patient's care. **(73)**

There are several laudable aspects to **EBP**. In particular, the idea that while the highest quality physical evidence should always be sought this should be balanced with what patients value and the decision-maker's clinical knowledge and experience. It also requires critical thinking about the evidence and its application and, done well, can constructively challenge established practice and policy, if there are improvements to be had.

Less positively, perhaps, time is needed to take this approach – nurses don't always have time to appraise the evidence or weigh up all the elements involved, especially in the here and now of emergency clinical situations and immediate ethical practice dilemmas. And there is no standard formula about how to balance **EBP's** three intertwined elements – which should be no surprise given how much healthcare decision-making relies on personal judgement.

For example, although there are grading systems for research evidence, which typically place randomised controlled trials as the most trusted, if the patient's values are in opposition to the evidence, which element do you choose to disregard? What the evidence says, and what matters to you as a clinician, may be less important to the patient. And when assessing the strength of research evidence, the nurse decision-maker must possess sufficient knowledge and skill to be able to discriminate wisely, which of course is itself a matter of personal judgement. But not every nurse has this experience and expertise. Nor is the best evidence always available to the practitioner.

How does **EBP** fare in Tom's case? As far as the research evidence is concerned it seems fairly clear that:

- E-cigarettes should never be assumed to be totally safe: they are not recommended for use by people who have never smoked, unless as an alternative to starting to smoke. (**74**)
- The emissions of e-cigarettes contain no tar and have less than one percent of the nitrosamines of tobacco smoke. (**75**)
- In normal use, aldehydes are less than ten percent of the levels found in tobacco smoke. (**76**)
- A complete replacement of smoking by e-cigarette use offers the nicotine user a dramatic decrease in the risk of serious diseases. (**77**)
- The option to switch to e-cigarettes should be considered by healthcare practitioners with patients with cancer who would otherwise continue to smoke. (**78**)

Given that Tom has terminal lung cancer, smokes heavily at home and enjoys it, has refused nicotine replacement therapy but has shown an interest in using an e-cigarette while in hospital, is it reasonable – according to the best evidence – to prevent him from using an e-cigarette in his room and grounds?

Our judgement is that this is not reasonable because there is no compelling evidence that e-cigarettes are harmful either to the vaper or to others. There may be a perceived risk to other patients who have respiratory issues such as asthma – but this is actually extremely low in this case since Tom is in a side room.

Nor does the hospital seem to be at risk from claims of negligence since harm is unforeseeable according to the best evidence we have to date.

There's currently no evidence to suggest that e-cigarettes would be harmful to Tom in the short term, and it's surely important to consider his quality of life in the short time he has left.

However, hospital policy is that he can't vape and must be clearly told that he can't. So, we see once again that the decision-making approach can inform the decision-maker up to a point; however, the actual decision – to try to prevent Tom from vaping or not – is up to the decision-maker, who may decide according to a wide range of reasons.

VALUES-BASED DECISION-MAKING

Values-based decision-making, or practice, is a further popular contemporary approach aimed at producing consistent decision-making. It's thought, for example, that if all health professionals value 'compassion' then, in circumstances which require compassion, each will be compassionate in the same way and, therefore, make the same practical decision.

But this understanding is incorrect, as various forms of research, including our own, clearly show.

OUR RESEARCH INTO VALUES

Between 2016 and 2018, with three colleagues, we carried out an online study using a dedicated Values Exchange website (**79**). The study was funded by the **UK Occupational Therapy Research Foundation**, which hoped to identify a consistent set of values that underpin occupational therapy practice in the UK. It was envisaged that the study's findings might be used to assist in 'values-based' recruitment, training and education, by making it possible to employ staff who share, or who could be taught to share, these values, and so make predictable decisions that all could rely upon.

Five commonplace, yet ethically challenging scenarios were created by a focus group of six occupational therapists, six service users and three researchers. All respondents were practising occupational therapists who volunteered to give and justify a decision about each scenario. Three of the scenarios were presented as online polls using a Likert Scale with **agree strongly**, **agree**, **disagree** and **disagree strongly** choices, plus unlimited free text commenting. The other two were Values Exchange 'cases', which offer respondents a wide range of pre-set ethical, social and practical concepts from which to choose, plus unlimited free text commenting. After submitting their views, respondents were able to comment on each other's responses in unlimited conversation threads – 553 unique responses were received over the five scenarios.

The hypothesis we tested was that occupational therapists' responses to ethically challenging situations would reveal a consistent set of values specific to the occupational therapy profession.

The results of our research refute the hypothesis. They show that while occupational therapists hold very general values in common, they do not always use the same specific values to make everyday practical choices. In fact, they often make conflicting decisions and justify them by referring to conflicting values. In particular:

- In each of the five scenarios, practising occupational therapists disagreed about what to do – there was never 100% agreement. In two cases there was considerable controversy (a 46% vs 54% split between agree and disagree in one and a 76% vs 24% split between agree and disagree in the other).
- Over all scenarios, respondents used a range of values and justifications. Both the stated values and the justifications for specific scenarios often conflicted between respondents.
- Respondents frequently referred to general values, like 'rights' and 'duty', to justify their choices, but as a group did not do so consistently. For example, while two respondents might both use 'rights' to justify their preferred choice of action, one might claim that the client has 'the right to choose' while the other might assert 'the right of the therapist' to override client choice.
- In situations where clients had expressed a clear choice, respondents tended to support client choice in some situations and yet deny client choice in similar situations; for example, where the client choice was perceived as 'costly of resources' or not in 'best interests'.
- Most respondents were explicitly conscious of their professional background and duties yet many offered personal reasons and justifications for their choices, expressing their own preferences rather than those of the professional body.
- General themes did emerge; for example, all respondents consistently expressed the desire to 'enable' their clients. However, the meaning of 'enabling' varied between respondents, and respondents often advanced directly conflicting practical ways of 'enabling'.

The full report of our research can be accessed here (**80**).

In brief, the funding body hoped and expected that the occupational therapists involved would draw similar conclusions to each other, and use the same values in the same way, so exhibiting a clear professional identity. But this is not what we found. Even when there was general agreement with a proposed course of action, the justifications and values used were varied. And when there was no agreement there were very clear conflicts of values.

This was true of all scenarios but is particularly striking in the following two:

SCENARIO 2.4: THE PERFECT WHEELCHAIR?

CATEGORIES: CLIENT PREFERENCE, RIGHTS, DUTY

George is a 14-year-old male with Cerebral Palsy, affecting all four limbs. George is known already to the Community Occupational Therapy Team.

You are a Paediatric Occupational Therapist and you have recently completed a home visit to George and his family – to reassess his current mobility equipment. It is found, after assessment, that the previous equipment is no longer suitable for George's current or future needs.

George's parents have recently visited (with George) a specialist show demonstrating new, state-of-the-art wheelchairs and equipment supplied by Naidex.

Both George and his parents have identified a chair which they feel would be both perfect for his current and future needs. George is also aware that this new chair will give him a degree of favourable status amongst his friends and peers, being high-tech and modern in appearance.

However, you're aware that there is a perfectly suitable chair available in the local community equipment stores, which Social Services would normally expect you to recommend. Social Services fund equipment for persons such as George. Although this chair is currently available, and resources are scarce, George is adamant that he does not want this chair as he sees it as old-fashioned and clunky.

Both George and his parents are insistent that they are only prepared to accept the high-tech chair.

What should you do?

It is proposed that you recommend the chair that George and his family have requested.

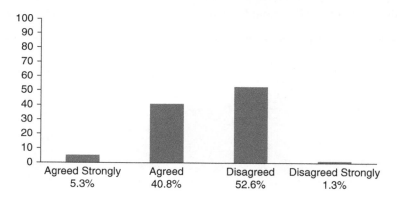

Figure 2.3   Scenario 2.4 Poll Results

—— SCENARIO 2.5: ILL OR NEEDY? ——

CATEGORIES: CLIENT PREFERENCE, RIGHTS, PROFESSIONAL DUTY

Andi is a 42-year-old female who suffers from Fibromyalgia – www.nhs.uk/Conditions/Fibromyalgia/Pages/Introduction.aspx – which was recently diagnosed following a long, drawn-out process.

Following this process, Andi has been left feeling very low, and desperate for assistance in both managing her condition and in others recognising her present and future needs.

(Continued)

After feeling that she has been 'written off' by many professionals during her diagnosis process, it has now been decided, after she asserted herself with her GP, that Andi be referred to Occupational Therapy (**OT**) for assessment. The manager of the **OT** department decides on a plan of action to send a newly qualified **OT** to see Andi, for an initial assessment of needs.

Andi wishes for equipment to help her, for example a stair lift, a walking aid, or a commode, but she is not exactly sure what she needs, and is not sure how the **OT** will feel, at this early stage, seeing her. Andi also feels that maybe having some equipment might make her feel more validated/affirmed by others, in her disability journey, being a disorder which is covert in nature and thus hidden from clear sight.

The **OT** visits Andi, where Andi is assertive in getting her perceived needs met. The **OT** feels hesitant, she does not think that Andi is yet in clinical need for equipment and wants to encourage Andi to remain as independent as possible without this equipment, for as long as is possible. The **OT** accepts that this equipment may be needed in the future if Andi's condition deteriorates. The **OT** feels that Andi is looking for a 'quick fix', which will solve her problems and feelings of frustration and vulnerability. Andi is adamant that she wants to exercise her choice in this matter.

The **OT** has some equipment in the car.

What do you think the OT should do? What would you do in these circumstances?

It is proposed that the Occupational Therapy fetches the equipment from the car.

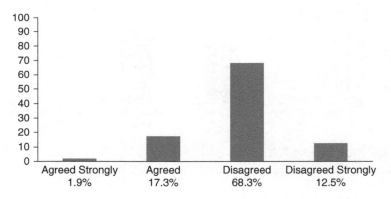

Figure 2.4   Scenario 2.5 Agreement or Disagreement with the proposal

While the circumstances of these two scenarios are very different, and there is inevitable 'framing' in how any scenario is presented, they share a central value, namely 'respect autonomy'. Both George and Andi have made very clear requests for support, and both are informed and resolute that they know what is in their best interests.

If the occupational therapist respondents really shared the same values-based outlook, then they ought to a) come to the same conclusions about each proposal and b) apply their value judgements consistently across scenarios that have the same central value in play. But we found that this was not the case.

Our respondents were not driven by a clear set of values – official or unofficial – rather they used their own personal judgements in social context.

Anyone who has been a part of any group of people knows that sooner or later human beings see things differently. These things can be matters of fact (is immigration a cause of greater unemployment or greater economic productivity?) or value (is cultural diversity an indication of a healthy social order or the erosion of 'our' values?) and often the two types of judgement are intertwined. Life is complex, and it's naive to imagine that broad generalisations (such as claims that 'professional values' can be standardised) can somehow override the complexities of personal judgement. For any life situation where there is no broadly agreed answer, some human beings will arrive at different conclusions and offer alternative justifications from other human beings, regardless of whether they are members of the same profession or other social grouping.

Our research shows that personal judgement, in context, drives occupational therapists' decision-making. Sometimes therapists agree about what to do and see circumstances in similar ways, and sometimes they disagree and see things differently. This is counter to the above hypothesis but entirely in keeping with commonsense experience of human decision-making.

EXAMPLES OF THE SAME RESPONDENTS USING DIFFERENT / CONFLICTING VALUES IN SIMILAR CIRCUMSTANCES

To falsify the study's hypothesis, we merely required contrary instances, of which there are many in our data. Below are examples of respondents using conflicting values in similar circumstances (all quotes presented as submitted to the Values Exchange).

Taking George's case we found numerous direct conflicts of values between occupational therapists. For example, Aly said:

I could not justify recommending something just because it is what the client and his parents want.

While Abigailo1 took exactly the opposite view:

We have a duty to suggest the other chair but it is down to the decision of George and his family.

Abigailo1 is also a typical example of a professional using conflicting values in similar situations. She agreed that the decision should be up to the client above (George), but for Andi she strongly disagreed:

It may be beneficial for Andi to receive intervention around health promotion and education around the condition. I would probably use that initial assessment getting to know Andi, what she previously liked doing – gaining trust and rapport. I would let her know that equipment is available but that this is something to explore next time. It may be that her psychological needs need to be met through psychology or counselling.

The therapist will respect George's choice even though there is a financial cost but will not respect Andi's even though there is no immediate cost. Autonomy is respected in one instance but not in another, and this contrast was found in many responses. Taking a similar line to Abigailo1, Joanna agreed with George's request:

> I have a professional duty to meet needs in a manner that is acceptable to the client.

But not Andi's:

> I may offer to bring some equipment at the next appointment to try if these were standard items from the loan store, but would be cautious about arranging a demo with a non-standard item if I was not sure I could justify the need for a special purchase. Alternatively I would direct her to the local disability resource centre if she was interested in private purchase or advise her of the 'cash contribution' if what she wanted was more expensive than a standard issue item.

Kimaliciamoxham22 also fitted this pattern:

> The other chair that is funding (sic) will meet George's physical needs yes, but what about his other needs? His emotional developmental needs? His new and emerging identity and role as he emerges into a teenager? That is why he wants a 'cool' and high tech chair. Image is and will be important to him. We are holistic OTs ... that is what we need to think about.

> I believe that Andi wants equipment because it will 'look' like she has an illness and therefore feel more 'validated/affirmed' by others as stated above. We are a very visual disability culture – if you don't see aids/adaptations then 'they don't have a disability'. The OT has assessed Andi as not clinically needing the equipment therefore same should not be administered at this stage.

In one case the respondent perceives a clear duty to meet the client's expressed need but not in the other case. Clearly, there is much more going on than pure values-based decision-making (the simple quantitative results illustrated above are enough on their own to show this).

The picture is more complex, when all responses are considered, as can be seen from the agree/disagree results above: 20 respondents would fetch the equipment for Andi.

SCOPE AND FRAMING

For any personal judgement, as part of the unique relationship between the **person** and the **circumstances** (elaborated in **Chapter Four**), it's important to consider two other facets: **scope** and **frame** – both of which are very well-known concepts in psychology.

'Scope' is simply how much of the circumstances are included in the judgement. Or to put it another way, how much of the circumstances are considered relevant by the person judging them. In some circumstances – emergency situations, for example, or in situations of high emotion (an intense marital row, for instance) the scope pretty much defines itself. In the emergency or within the row, the person's attention is mostly or entirely focused on just that, and nothing else, and there is little or no conscious choice about how much of the circumstances to include. However, in non-emergency situations – in everyday healthcare situations, for example – the scope is usually mostly defined by the person judging. Is this just about the patient directly in front of me? Or is it about all patients on the ward? Or is it about all patients and staff on the ward? Is this situation about patients now or about future patients too? Is it about the hospital? Is it about my role as a nurse? Is it about my work–life balance? Is it about helping me get promotion? A new job? How the scope is defined depends on some balance between what the person considers important and the external circumstances that are in play.

'Frame' is less about the circumstances and more about how the person it concerns sees, interprets and colours what is going on. It's really about how the person views, or is able to view the situation. It's about what the judge brings to the situation – it's about how the person's perspective affects the relationship between her and the situation and, therefore, affects her judgement.

We can see this framing effect in many of our scenarios. For example, in **Scenario 6.1 (Chapter Six)** we present an incident involving a nurse, Carol, who has taken food from the patients' food trolley for her lunch. Is this a good or bad thing?

How you see her – how you begin to judge the whole situation in fact – as you enter the Staff Room and notice she is eating the patients' food, depends on many factors that you bring to the situation. Seeing Carol eating the food – whoever sees it – is not a neutral event. It's a combination of you and the situation.

Consider how the situation actually changes (you could say 'appears different', but we think it actually changes) as personal factors change. Is Carol your friend? Do you dislike her? Is she your rival? Has she tried to help you in the past? Has she tried to damage you? Have you done what she is doing? Are you in charge of the ward? Do you need to exert authority? Are you a kind person, or are you vindictive? Do you see your job as only to help the people you see in front of you, or do you see yourself as a guardian of resources? Do you think you are bound by a law? By a clause in an ethical code? Are you fearful you will be punished if you don't report Carol? Or couldn't you care less? Whatever the case, it will make a significant difference to the reality in front of both of you (and of course Carol will be making her own personal judgements, just as you are).

In this case, as in the majority of cases, scope and frame blur together. For example, if you think of your role as a guardian of resources, you will likely consider the scope of this situation broadly, and perhaps think that you need to act to avoid wide and long-term negative consequences, were this to become common practice amongst staff. But if you couldn't care less – or if you think how other nurses act is none of your business – you may not even notice what Carol is doing.

PERSONAL OR PROFESSIONAL JUDGEMENT?

The occupational therapy project raised an interesting and often confused question of definition. It is very common to hear reference to 'clinical' or 'professional' judgement in the health and nursing literature, for example the NMC Code states:

... all of the professions we regulate exercise professional judgement and are accountable for their work. (**28**)

The implication is that somehow these forms of judgement are more substantial or perhaps more objective than 'personal judgement'. However, it is quite clear to us that it's arbitrary to divide judgement up in this way. There are no separate categories of human judgement – there is simply judgement made by people in whatever role – professional or otherwise – they have at any given time.

The nurse exercising 'clinical' or 'professional' judgement is not exercising a special form of judgement, she is exercising her judgement as a person in the particular circumstances she has to deal with at the time. That's all.

As McShea has perceptively noted:

Clinical judgment involves the personal orientation, the ethical framework of the one making the decision. Whatever judgment is ultimately made carries with it the burden of the maker's personal ethical approach to life, to the nature of man and finally his approach to the world at large. Clinical judgment is inseparable from ethics. (**81**)

This came as a surprise to the funders of our occupational therapy study, who clearly expected to find a) that occupational therapists as a professional body hold the same values and b) that these values would to some extent be different from the values of other professions.

On the face of it, it does seem *prima facie* reasonable to believe that working in a particular context – for example as a nurse for twenty years – will have a major impact and affect the professionals' perceptions and choices. And this is true, but to a much lesser extent than is commonly believed. There are so many and so varied other factors in play – life is just more complicated than this.

WHAT ABOUT TOM?

Using values-based practice everything hinges, of course, on the values you adopt and what they mean to you. Like the other approaches, things become rather vague very quickly.

One value that is often said to be central to good nursing is 'compassion'. Say you decide that this is what is driving you, you can nevertheless use it to justify allowing or forbidding Tom to vape. On the one hand, he has little time left to live, so it would be 'compassionate' to let him use the e-cigarette; on the other, it is possible that it might irritate his lungs and that this would cause guilt to his family.

THE FOUR PRINCIPLES

The 'four principles of biomedical ethics' are set out in various editions of *Principles of Biomedical Ethics*, by Beauchamp and Childress. The text has been revised and updated over the years but continues to argue, essentially, that it's possible to make 'ethical decisions' by applying only 'four principles'. **(82)**

These principles are:

1. Beneficence (the obligation to provide benefits and balance benefits against risks)
2. Non-maleficence (the obligation to avoid the causation of harm)
3. Respect for autonomy (the obligation to respect the decision-making capacities of autonomous persons)
4. Justice (obligations of fairness in the distribution of benefits and risks)

By using them, either singly or in combination, a health carer is supposed to be able to give a satisfactory answer to any moral problem she comes across in her work. Beauchamp admits that she may need 'additional interpretation and specification', and perhaps further rules such as 'don't kill' and 'tell the truth', but fundamentally the four principles, on their own, are supposed to be enough for all practical, moral deliberation in healthcare.

Many commentators – including one of us (David) – have severely criticised the four-principles approach as a 'mantra of principles', dogma repeated with little reflection or analysis. The philosophers Gert and Clouser **(83)**, for example, point out that the 'four principles' are little more than checklists or headings and as such cannot produce specific guidelines for moral conduct. There's no theory or justification for the principles (why these principles and not others?), and in the real world the principles will always compete in difficult circumstances, yet Beauchamp and Childress offer no advice about how to deal consistently with either theoretical or practical conflict, because this would require reason and action beyond the principles themselves.

Just think about any real case – or any scenario in this book – and try to apply nothing other than the 'four principles' to solve it. It's almost immediately obvious that a) which principle or combination of principles to use and b) what each principle means in context and c) how you justify your choices, are all matters of personal judgement.

A research project entitled: *The four principles: Can they be measured and do they predict ethical decision making?* is highly instructive. Its author, Katie Page, summarises:

> This study test[ed] whether [the four] principles can be quantitatively measured on an individual level, and then subsequently if they are used in the decision mak-ing process when individuals are faced with ethical dilemmas .... Four scenarios, which involved conflicts between the ... principles, were presented to participants who then made judgements about the ethicality of the action in the scenario, and their intentions to act in the same manner if they were in the situation .... On average, individuals [had] a significant preference for non-maleficence over the other principles, however, and perhaps counter-intuitively, this preference (did) not seem to relate to applied ethical judgements in specific ethical dilemmas ... **People state they value these medical ethical principles but they do not actually seem to use them directly in the decision making process.** (Bold ours) **(84)**

In other words, while Beauchamp and Childress' four 'ethical principles' may seem meaningful in the abstract – who could disagree in principle with the desire to 'minimise harm' for example? – in practice, real-world decision-making is massively more complex, and profoundly affected by the prevailing circumstances, as we found in our own values-based decision-making research discussed above, and as we further explain in **Chapter Four.**

As Page says:

> ... the weights elicited with abstract questions about the principles (independently from contextual information) have no predictive power to explain the partici- pants' choices in specific scenarios ... which suggest(s) that the application of principles in scenarios is not consistent because the principles are not related to ethical judgments ... situational information seems to be of greater importance.

This is a devastatingly important finding. We do not wish to be harsh, but at a stroke it condemns library shelves full of works on 'ethical principles', ethical codes, buzzword checklists like the **6Cs**, and any other abstract theoretical assertion, to the nearest skip. Just as with 'values-based recruitment', in the abstract people may say they have fundamental values they would apply in any situation, but as soon as it comes to real decisions we immediately forget these abstract ideals. Instead we work out what to do dependent on the circumstances in front of us, and *how we think and feel about them at that particular time*. This cannot be overstated – hence our use of italics: personal judgement is always and constantly required, and it never occurs in the abstract. We bring ourselves, as we are at the time, to the circumstances, as we perceive them at that time, and then, having created a unique reality, we make our choices. (**85**)

As we saw in our occupational therapy research – and as we explain in **Chapter Four** – contrary to most people's expectations, people's judgements are simply not always consistent. Just as in the **Train Journey** in **Chapter Three**, we affect the circumstances and they affect us in a dynamic relationship. Therefore, trying to 'lay down the ethical law' with 'ethical commandments' and static 'principles' is not only completely pointless and ineffective, it's a corruption of how we actually think and act. Teaching 'the four principles' and similar unempirical dogma as if it is truth could, therefore, be considered a form of moral and intellectual abuse.

Given this, we conclude that the 'four principles' are irrelevant to Tom's case. You can of course try to use them if you wish. However, it will be you doing the thinking, not the 'four principles'.

NURSING ETHICS

There is a considerable literature about nursing ethics, to which one of us (David) has contributed in various publications.

There is some debate about whether 'nursing ethics' is a distinct field of study, but in our view this hardly matters. 'Medical ethics', 'nursing ethics', 'engineering ethics', 'professional ethics' and so on are all obviously related. The main differences are the case studies and examples the various textbooks and articles use.

Typically, texts on 'nursing ethics' provide an introduction to the terminology. For example, most attempt to differentiate between key terms: 'ethics and morality', 'rights and virtues', 'facts and values', 'consequences and duties' and so on. They explain that different schools of thought favour one or more of these ideas over the others, and point out the pros and cons of each.

There is usually a sizeable discussion of the differences between 'consequentialism' and 'deontology', concepts most often gleaned from introductory courses on moral philosophy, or from the many other professional ethics text in circulation. These are typically introduced as distinct technical terms and approaches. Readers are informed, for example, that a strict 'consequentialist' will judge the morality of a choice or action on the outcome alone, regardless of good or bad intent (an ethical decision will produce 'good' results – benefits of some kind – and an unethical choice will produce 'bad' consequences). Whereas a strict 'deontologist' will always do what they consider right on principle, regardless of the consequences – for example, a person of this persuasion may think it ethical always to tell the truth, even if to do so will cause avoidable harm (**86**).

It is also common to find 'the four principles' referred to as 'fundamental', without any explanation of why this should be the case (**87**). It is just accepted that they are, even though they have been selected from a wide range of other alternative principles, and are vaguely expressed and open to broad interpretation.

After the introductory remarks, case studies are introduced and assessed from the perspective of the different 'ethical theories'. Often, because there are so many different perspectives, the analyses tend to become both lengthy and dense, which can make matters confusing for students, who really have no idea which of the many theories they should choose themselves.

One striking feature of all the texts in this genre is that while they present useful and challenging case studies, their authors rarely say what they would do in the circumstances, leaving the reader stranded. For example:

> [Ethical choices] may involve conflict between duty to the patient and duty to society. Ethical conflicts may also involve the clash between two ethical duties (such as the duty to respect and promote autonomy and the duty to benefit the patient). They may involve tensions between the ethical positions of professional and religious groups to which the nurse feels loyalty. They may involve tension between the rights of patients and the nurse's self-interest and welfare. (**86**)

They may then go on to illustrate the tensions with case studies but make no attempt to resolve them.

In some ways this is understandable since the purpose of such books is mainly to introduce concepts and example problems, but it is also extremely frustrating. Such texts make it completely obvious that everything ultimately depends on personal judgement, but do not examine the process of judgement, which is plainly required to: a) identify that there is an ethical problem; b) identify different ethical approaches to the problem (for example, is this issue about 'individual rights' or 'the public interest'?); c) identify the 'ethical tensions'; d) choose which ethical approach to apply; e) define the approach in context; and f) apply the approach to reach a resolution.

Because of this common trend in the literature, we recommend reading books on 'nursing ethics' sparingly, and with a focus on the case studies. We do not believe that real-life decision-making proceeds according to strict theoretical distinctions; it is a much more personal process than this, and can and is continually done by millions of people without explicit knowledge of ethical theory.

This is not to say that 'nursing ethics' is of no use. Recognising the different theories can, to some extent, help you become more self-aware. For example, you might find yourself drawn to ways of deciding based on 'rights' or 'equality' or 'creating autonomy' (which we tend to favour ourselves (**20**)), and this will tell you something about yourself, your preferences and a little of what influences your own judgements. You might then ask yourself what it is about you, as a person, that causes you to feel this way.

In Tom's case, you can clearly use nursing ethics to argue that he should be able to vape (saying it is his 'human right', for example) and that he should not (saying that it infringes the 'human rights' of others, or using literally tens of alternative reasons based on one ethical theory or another).

INTUITION

Intuition is often said to be an important aspect of nurses' decision-making, as well as being a familiar feature of life in general:

> Most of us experience 'gut feelings' we can't explain, such as instantly loving – or hating – a new property when we're househunting or the snap judgements we make on meeting new people. Now researchers at Leeds say these feelings – or intuitions – are real and we should take our hunches seriously.

> According to a team led by Professor Gerard Hodgkinson of the Centre for Organisational Strategy, Learning and Change at Leeds University Business School, intuition is the result of the way our brains store, process and retrieve information on a subconscious level and so is a real psychological phenomenon which needs further study to help us harness its potential.

> There are many recorded incidences where intuition prevented catastrophes and cases of remarkable recoveries when doctors followed their gut feelings. Yet science has historically ridiculed the concept of intuition, putting it in the same box as parapsychology, phrenology and other 'pseudoscientific' practices.

> Through analysis of a wide range of research papers examining the phenomenon, the researchers conclude that intuition is the brain drawing on past experiences and external cues to make a decision – but one that happens so fast the reaction is at a non-conscious level. All we're aware of is a general feeling that something is right or wrong.

> 'People usually experience true intuition when they are under severe time pressure or in a situation of information overload or acute danger, where conscious analysis of the situation may be difficult or impossible,' says Professor Hodgkinson.

> He cites the recorded case of a Formula One driver who braked sharply when nearing a hairpin bend without knowing why – and as a result avoided hitting a pile-up of cars on the track ahead, undoubtedly saving his life.

'The driver couldn't explain why he felt he should stop, but the urge was much stronger than his desire to win the race,' explains Professor Hodgkinson. 'The driver underwent forensic analysis by psychologists afterwards, where he was shown a video to mentally relive the event. In hindsight he realised that the crowd, which would have normally been cheering him on, wasn't looking at him coming up to the bend but was looking the other way in a static, frozen way. That was the cue. He didn't consciously process this, but he knew something was wrong and stopped in time.'

Prof Hodgkinson believes that all intuitive experiences are based on the instantaneous evaluation of such internal and external cues – but does not speculate on whether intuitive decisions are necessarily the right ones.

'Humans clearly need both conscious and non-conscious thought processes, but it's likely that neither is intrinsically "better" than the other,' he says.

As a Chartered occupational psychologist, Professor Hodgkinson is particularly interested in the impact of intuition within business, where many executives and managers claim to use intuition over deliberate analysis when a swift decision is required. 'We'd like to identify when business people choose to switch from one mode to the other and why – and also analyse when their decision is the correct one. By understanding this phenomenon, we could then help organisations to harness and hone intuitive skills in their executives and managers.' (**88, 89**)

As illustrated by **Spectra 1** and **2**, some scholars prefer objective, evidence-based approaches, while others see special value in hunches and 'non-rational' insights. In the end it seems both poles have their place:

The strength of our intuition often urges us to do something more for the patient. When we as nurses report our intuitions, subjective feelings are often at odds with the objective signs and symptoms. Nurses have made great strides in recognizing, analysing and teaching concepts related to logical, rational decision-making. It is imperative, however, also to recognize and teach the concepts related to the intuitive and precognitive components of making decisions in clinical practice. (**90**)

In recent years, Daniel Kahneman and Gary Klein have extensively debated the nature and value of intuition. Both are academic psychologists. Kahneman favours scientific, overtly rational ways of decision-making (though his views have mellowed over time) while Klein says such precision fails to reflect the way people actually make decisions (**91, 92**).

Kahneman claims that countless psychological experiments show that human beings overrate our decision-making powers. We see a blurred or distorted version of reality and, therefore, make less effective decisions than we would were we to use scientifically tested protocols and formulae. Kahneman gives many examples, including the 'halo effect', under which we form a superficial impression of a person based on limited experience, which then influences how we feel about other aspects of their character about which we know nothing at all – 'he's nice' therefore he must also be 'smart'.

Kahneman sees our reverence for 'intuition' and 'intuitive people' as a delusion. He argues that when it comes to 'intuition vs formulas', formulae win hands down. He observes that when you compare:

> ... clinical predictions based on the subjective impressions of trained professionals [with] statistical predictions made by combining a few scores or ratings according to a rule ... about 60% of the studies show significantly better accuracy for the algorithms .... The other comparisons scored a draw in accuracy but a tie is tantamount to a win for the statistical rules, which are normally much less expensive to use than expert judgement.

Examples of rule-based predicted outcomes abound: longevity of cancer patients, length of hospital stays, prospects of success for new businesses, evaluation of credit risks for banks, winners of football games, future prices of Bordeaux wine ...

> ... in every case the accuracy of the experts was matched or succeeded by a simple algorithm ...

In his wine example the formula included only three features of weather to predict:

> ... a particular property at a particular age ... the average temperature over the summer growing season, the amount of rain at harvest time, and the total rainfall during the previous winter .... His formula forecasts future prices much more accurately than the prices of young wines do.

For the same reasons, bookmakers don't go out of business. They're the perfect example of the supremacy of algorithms vs human guesswork – the wisest and most informed punter may win sometimes but with even simple rules on their side the bookies will always win out in due course.

Kahneman even goes so far as to say that:

> ... it is unethical to rely on intuitive judgments for important decisions if an algorithm is available that will make fewer mistakes.

He uses this example of a 'mistaken intuition':

> ... the reliance on a heuristic produces a predictable bias in judgments. For example, I recently came to doubt my long-held impression that adultery is more common among politicians than among physicians or lawyers. I had even come up with explanations for that 'fact', including the aphrodisiac effect of power and the temptations of life away from home. I eventually realised that the transgressions of politicians are much more likely to be reported than the transgressions of lawyers and doctors. My intuitive impression could be due entirely to journalists' choices of topics ...

To be fair this isn't really an argument against intuition. It's merely an example of the importance of being careful about one's assumptions. Kahneman's 'intuition' was sloppy thinking, not a demonstration of a fundamental flaw in the process of well-grounded intuition.

For Kahneman, the default position about human judgement is that it's likely to be mistaken. Klein, on the other hand, rejects this point of view because it's based upon 'artificial tasks assigned in laboratory settings', which has the effect of making people seem 'biased and unskilled'. Instead, Klein developed the concept of 'naturalistic decision-making' (or **NDM**), which views people as 'inherently skilled', given sufficient experience in their field. Klein spent years watching fire commanders, fighter pilots, paramedics and others making 'split second decisions on the job', which led him to conclude that 'the expert decision-maker who behaves according to rational models' is rather a myth.

When he began his research, Klein expected his subjects to use systematic, rational, analytic methods, comparing possible options and selecting the most beneficial or effective:

> ... a deliberated choice between two or more options ... a systematic process of evaluation.

In fact, Klein discovered that expert decision-makers do not go through a mechanism of 'comparative evaluation' – there just isn't time to do this:

> In fact, they were using a different strategy altogether.

Klein explains:

> It was not that commanders were refusing to compare options: rather they did not have to compare options ... the commanders could come up with a good course of action from the start .... Even when faced with a complex situation, the com- manders could see it as familiar and know how to react ... Their experience let them identify a reasonable reaction as the first they considered, so they did not bother thinking of others. They were not being perverse. They were being skilful. We now call this strategy RECOGNITION-PRIMED DECISION MAKING ... fireground commanders use the power of mental simulation, running the action through in their minds. If they spot a potential problem, like the rescue harness not working well, they move onto the next option.

Before he looked closely, Klein believed it would be novices who jumped impulsively to the first option they could think of but:

> ... now it seemed that it was the experts who could generate a single course of action, while novices needed to compare different approaches.

Kahneman also accepts that this is important. To be a good intuitive decision-maker you need to have spent many hours (possibly thousands) analysing, reconstructing and experimenting with the phenomenon you wish to become expert in:

> ... after thousands of hours of practice ... chess masters are able to read a chess situation at a glance.

So, where do they disagree?

> We eventually concluded that our disagreement was due in part to the fact that we had different experts in mind. Klein had spent much of his time with fireground commanders, clinical nurses and other professionals who have real expertise. I had spent more time thinking about clinicians, stock pickers and political scientists trying to make unsupportable long-term forecasts.

Both Kahneman and Klein have a point. Kahneman worries about 'pseudo experts who have no idea that they do not know what they are doing' while Klein is concerned that over-reliance on algorithms undervalues the power of human perception.

One obvious implication for healthcare/nursing education is to build experience through testable practice as early and as much as possible.

Patricia Benner was an early advocate of intuition – or 'tacit knowledge' – in nursing. The term 'tacit' knowledge was first described by Michael Polanyi, a scientist and philosopher, who pointed out that '... we can know more than we can tell' (**93**). For Polanyi, 'tacit knowledge' is a form of 'unconscious knowing' – acquired through practice and experience rather than through language. Tacit knowledge is not ultimately mysterious, but it is difficult to communicate because it forms and grows as the result of countless individual experiences (**94**).

Like Klein, Benner sees that expert nurses develop skills and understanding in patient care over time through a multitude of experiences, in addition to their having a necessary educational base.

She describes five levels of nursing experience – well-grounded intuition grows steadily as the nurse advances through these levels:

- Novice
- Advanced beginner
- Competent
- Proficient
- Expert (**95**)

This, of course, does not mean that we always see patterns correctly – even as experts – or that we see the best patterns from all the possible patterns we are looking at.

However, some things are obvious where intuition is concerned:

- There can be no intuition without experience.
- Any intuitive insight must identify a pattern (for example, intuiting but not directly knowing that it will rain soon).
- If there are patterns then it is possible to test the intuition – does this pattern really exist or is it a delusion of some kind?
- There can be many possible patterns to intuit – deciding which is the right one can also be an intuitive process, or it may be based on overt analysis of evidence, or on some combination.

INTUITION IN NURSE EDUCATION

This paper reports a fascinating example in nursing (**96**): 181 nurses who cared for neonates in mother–infant and neonatal intensive care units (**NICU**) were asked to complete an email survey to ascertain which physiological and behavioural indicators were most often associated with neonatal sepsis.

Participants identified six signs and symptoms. Two were physiological and four were behavioural. The researchers discovered that recognition of these indicators was not related to the level of nursing education but was instead associated with working in the NICU. Seventy-three per cent of participants reported that they suspected that newborns were septic before the formal, clinical evaluation and diagnosis of septicaemia.

Overall, we agree that intuition is a vital part of healthcare, and is usually under-emphasised in nurse education. However, there are three provisos:

1. We may intuit the wrong or unhelpful pattern.
2. We may focus on the pattern we feel is best but our focus may obscure more useful patterns.
3. In situations of social or ethical complexity (as in our scenarios) – unlike in most clinical care – there are no RIGHT patterns to intuit. The best we can do is recall openly – or intuit rapidly – that given this sort of circumstance (X) then this sort of response (Y) may well be best (**97, 98, 99, 100, 101, 102, 103**).

WHAT ABOUT TOM?

It's not easy to see how intuition could help in Tom's case. Klein's notion of 'recognition primed decision-making' does have some relevance, though cannot detect 'the right answer'.

If we were to compare a novice decision-maker in this area – for example a student nurse on placement – with a seasoned nurse, then the latter would be more likely at least to have a deeper understanding of what matters most. She would perhaps be better placed to intuit Tom's level of distress, to read his body language, to know what alternative options to suggest and how to suggest them, to know what to say to the family and to know – without thinking – how best to defuse any awkward situations that might arise.

THE ETHICAL GRID

Many years ago, one of us (David) came up with a colourful way of thinking about ethical problems. This method used a Grid of concepts from which the decision-maker could select those which best explained and justified her decision (see **104**).

The Ethical Grid has been fairly widely used in ethics teaching in healthcare and is extensively explained in other publications, which interested readers are invited to explore.

There are several versions of the Grid; printed, made out of wooden blocks, and as software on the Values Exchange. This is how it appeared in *Ethics: The Heart of Health Care*, in which it was first introduced **(20)**.

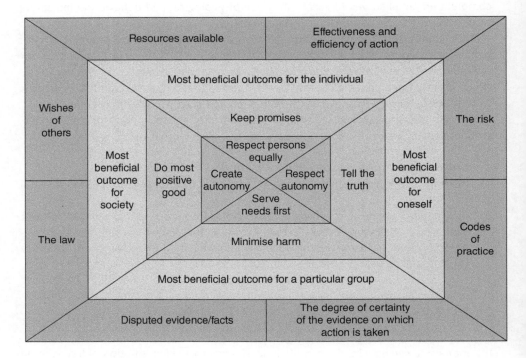

Figure 2.5   The Ethical Grid

The Grid is designed to support systematic, balanced decision-making. It includes a range of practical and philosophical considerations, which the user may select and define in order to justify a specific decision.

The Grid is arranged in a square, with four levels, three containing 4 tiles and one containing 8. The four levels are: practicalities (8 tiles), consequences, duties and purpose. Simply put, the idea is that, to be balanced, any real-world decision should include tiles from at least two levels and in healthcare all four, and that the choice of tile – what each means in context – is up to the decision-maker.

There are several ways to use the Ethical Grid, but the most common is to use it to justify a practical proposal. In order to do this, the user visually scans the Grid, as much as possible with an open mind, and chooses a tile that somehow 'springs out' or resonates as most relevant in the situation. She must then think about what that tile means to her, in the context of the proposal, and may then consider other tiles, if she wishes. The goal is to select a few tiles – say three to five – she's defined and selected as most significant in the circumstances. These are the concepts and definitions she will use to explain and justify her decision.

Two aspects of the Grid are especially relevant here. These are, first, the fact that the Grid is merely a support to decision-making – it cannot possibly be used without subjective, personal judgement; and second, that it contains 20 concepts. On the Grid, 'law', 'risk' and 'evidence', for example, are not decisive concepts, rather they need to be balanced with other ideas, and need not be used at all if the decision-maker does not see them as important in the circumstances, or believes other tiles are more important.

This contrasts, for example, with 'risk-management' initiatives that assume an imperative to reduce or avoid risks, regardless of other practical and ethical considerations, and instructions that a nurse **must** use the **NMC** code regardless of her own views.

The Ethical Grid anticipates our theory of personal judgement. It was specifically designed to be used in the 'grey area' of healthcare (see **Chapter Three**). Different people can and do use the Grid to come up with different solutions – and this is not only a good thing, but it reflects the way the world actually is.

This said, like the 'four principles', the Grid is artificial and contrived. The initial idea was that users would be able to choose concepts as they occurred to them, intuitively orienting their thinking to those concepts that struck them as most important, rather than decide in a linear way, so as to reflect the way we actually think. In practice, however, people rarely use the Grid to make actual decisions – in real life we don't think as analytically and presciently as this.

The Grid works well in teaching sessions and seminars – highlighting some of the theoretical complexity of decision-making – but just like the other technical approaches we set out in this chapter, it underestimates the power and mystery of the human factor.

In Tom's case, yet again the Grid can be used to argue for and against taking the e-cigarette from him. To argue for its removal, a decision-maker might choose 'wishes of others', 'risk' and 'minimise harm'. To be plausible in taking this stance, the decision-maker could not refer to 'health risks' or 'physical harm', as we discuss above, but she could point to the risk of disputes and arguments amongst staff, disruption to the smooth-running of the ward, and the consensus amongst staff to follow official policy. To argue against taking the e-cigarette from Tom, a decision-maker might use 'evidence', 'do most positive good', 'most beneficial outcome for the individual' (Tom) and 'respect autonomy'.

SUMMARY OF CHAPTER TWO

1) This chapter has introduced ten standard approaches to decision-making that are frequently used in nursing and healthcare
2) Most of these sit to the left of the decision-making spectrum
3) In order to use one or more of the approaches a personal choice has to be made
4) There are no absolute rules either for deciding which approach to use or how to apply whatever particular approach or approaches you use
5) We use the case of a terminally ill life-long smoker to illustrate the importance and limitations of each approach

6) Each, sooner or later, reaches a limit at which point personal judgement is required
7) At present, personal judgement remains a largely mysterious entity
8) We try to understand more about it in **Chapter Four**

CHAPTER TWO EXERCISES

Having read **Chapter Two** you may like to attempt the following exercises, to reinforce your learning:

1. Describe the advantages and disadvantages of **two** different approaches to nursing decision-making introduced in this chapter
2. Apply each approach either to a scenario in **Chapters Five**, **Six** or **Seven** or to real-life circumstances you have encountered or read about
3. For each, identify and demonstrate the point at which personal judgement is necessary
4. For each, use your personal judgement to find a solution you feel is most justifiable
5. Explain both your feelings and your reasoning

CHAPTER 3

MYTHS AND FACTS ABOUT HEALTHCARE DECISION-MAKING

AIMS

This chapter has the following aims:

1) To describe six myths and six facts about decision-making in nursing and healthcare
2) To offer a story about a hypothetical train journey as a metaphor for our everyday experience, and to illustrate how complex and uncertain even the simplest healthcare interactions are
3) To illustrate that the widespread desire to minimise personal judgement in order to provide standardised nursing and healthcare is unrealistic and unachievable
4) To suggest that accepting the power and necessity of personal judgement in nursing and healthcare is a mature and professional approach that should be embraced rather than feared

LEARNING OUTCOMES

When you have read and worked through this chapter you should be able to:

1) Appreciate and be able to explain the six myths and facts
2) Reflect on and discuss the myths and facts and show, with examples, how they relate to nursing and healthcare
3) Give examples of nursing and healthcare decision-making from the 'grey area' described in **Myth One**
4) State and explain whether or not you agree with our account of the myths and facts

In writing this book we have come to realise how ignorant we are about decision-making. By 'we' we do not mean just the two of us, we mean all of us. Because we have such impressive science and technology in the modern world – and not least in healthcare – it's tempting to think that this level of genuine knowledge and application extends equally into all our spheres of interest: that just as we can transplant organs, send messages and images at the speed of light, and construct phenomenal skyscrapers and bridges, so we assume we understand what makes us tick as human beings. But we don't. Genius in one thing never guarantees genius in anything else. In fact, it's more likely to lead to blindness.

We make most of our judgements unaware we are making them. We are strangely untroubled by this. If we do think about our thinking we tend to assume we're more in control of it than we really are, and we sustain this fiction with a set of myths, which most of us rarely question.

We explain these myths in this chapter. We do not claim to be unarguably right; indeed, we may well be mistaken in all that we say. The myths – and their counter-balancing facts – are merely an expression of our current, very limited understanding of nursing and healthcare decision-making.

We present the myths in the context of nursing and healthcare; however, they are equally relevant to any other profession and are, we believe, a feature of life we should all reflect on, if we are to understand ourselves and the world a little more deeply.

To give a life context for the myths and facts, first consider the following story about a simple, imaginary train journey. We present it as a metaphor for the entire book.

THE TRAIN JOURNEY

Imagine a train carriage. In the carriage there are 50 or so people, of many ages and backgrounds. Each has a different seat, so each has a different view of the carriage and the landscape outside.

Some are sitting with strangers, some are sitting with acquaintances, some are sitting with friends and some are sitting with people they know but don't get on with, or just don't like the look of. Each passenger has her own thoughts and memories and each boarded the train today from different life contexts. Some were kissed goodbye by partners they're happy with, some weren't kissed, a couple of them had just had a row, some are doing well, some are unhappy, some are ill, some are stressed, several are wondering what in hell's name they're doing here – it's a typical train compartment on a typical day.

The train is crowded. Some passengers are forced to stand. Out of the blue, two of them start to argue. One's a man – he's noticeably overweight, with rolls of flesh bulging under his tight-fitting shirt. The other's a woman with a small toddler. There are two other young children nearby – they're becoming upset by the kerfuffle and start to cry. The large man is sitting down, occupying a double seat. He refuses to relinquish it for the woman and child, even though she's asked him pleasantly and is obviously stressed and harassed. He says he's disabled by his weight. Not his fault. He needs both seats more than she does and he can't move over because of his size.

As events unfold, each passenger in the carriage has an ethical/social/practical problem to solve – it doesn't really matter what label you give it. And each has a unique set of influences they bring with them – a unique 'set of baggage' if you like. Each passenger has a different life history, personality, age, job, friends, different knowledge, different skills, fears, hopes, expectations and current life circumstances. Each passenger is unique – which means that each is bound to see, and so define, the situation differently, possibly very differently.

For some, the incident may be trivial – perhaps they're absorbed with their own thoughts and either don't notice or don't much care. Whereas for others it may be very significant – perhaps one is a disability rights advocate, perhaps another experienced a similar incident as a child, and was traumatised by it.

(Continued)

Apart from the few people in the carriage who seem oblivious to the circumstances, and for whom there is therefore no situation, each person will – consciously or unconsciously – define the situation in their own way. For some, the incident may just spring up and disappear once it's resolved, and never be remembered. While others may see it as part of a long-standing, systemic disregard for ticket-purchasing railway customers forced to endure daily overcrowding – a social issue, a political issue, a triumph of the profit motive over respectful regard for others.

One passenger is a policewoman, who has good knowledge of the law and the consequences of breaking it. Another is a photographer with a video camera, another's a judo expert, one's a doctor, one's a philosopher, another's a counsellor, two of them are local journalists, three are retired, one passenger is travelling home after receiving chemotherapy.

Because of who they are they will personally experience the train journey in different ways. It may be that the policewoman or the counsellor will try to intervene, because they're used to doing so, though in different ways – the policewoman may instruct while the counsellor may try to broker a compromise. Or it may be that the photographer welcomes the conflict and wants more of it, since it will provide good footage for her YouTube channel. Or one of the journalists may sniff a good story. Simply put, the passengers' conflict may be judged to be a positive or negative situation dependent upon the person observing it.

Now the guard arrives. He has a rule-book. It says that if there's a request to give up a seat for a disabled person or a mother with child then that must be consented to, but of course this does not solve the present problem, because both the man and the mother arguably have an equal claim.

The woman with child tells the guard, 'There are two of us.' But the man counters, 'Having a child's normal. It was your choice. I'm disabled.'

The guard is troubled and unsure what to do. Then someone fires up an e-cigarette in the carriage. Relieved to find circumstances where there's a definite rule, the guard quickly announces that this is not allowed, and would the passenger please desist. But the passenger simply takes a deep drag on the e-cigarette, produces a doctor's letter, and says it's a prescription – medication for pain relief for his increasingly severe MS. If he doesn't use it every few minutes the pain becomes disablingly severe, so he must be allowed.

Suddenly, the man with the double seat starts to hold his chest. He's sweating. He collapses in an apparent faint. Two nurses move forward. They're friends. The first nurse reaches in her bag for a bottle of aspirin and some water. The second nurse holds her back. 'No. Stop. You don't know. It's too risky,' she says. The first nurse turns to her. 'But we can't just turn our backs. He needs help. I'm going to try CPR. I'm trained.' The second nurse rapidly counters. 'No. No. Anything could happen,' she replies.

For a moment it's as if the carriage is frozen. Still. Then the child starts to choke. His mother screams. She tries to open his mouth. He's got his lolly stuck. Help. Help.

Immediately, and as one, both nurses turn away from the man, and help the child. The first gives back blows, which don't work. The other skilfully administers abdominal thrusts. The lolly pops out. The child cries and clings to his mother …

We don't like to think of ourselves as passengers, at the mercy of factors beyond our control (which is one reason so many people prefer their private cars over public transport). We like to think we can make independent choices, regardless of what's happening around us. But human existence is not like this. To some extent we can choose which train to get on, but once we're on it we're very obviously subject to an array of forces over which we have no authority whatsoever.

In life, at work and play, we're all part of a ceaseless, incredibly varied and fascinating journey – a mystery-tour in a capricious vehicle to a destination none of us knows and none of us has chosen. Most of our fellow-passengers are strangers to us. They get on. We may interact, we may not. They get off. The train moves on. The scenery changes. New people board. They make choices. We make choices. Things change. We change things. Things change us. It's a drama. A perpetual work of art with infinite perspectives.

There are no protocols and no definitive ethical guidance for life's train journeys. There are no neutral experiences on the train. The passengers are not separate from the journey's events. They affect the events and the events affect them. Precisely how this will happen is always unpredictable, for any journey.

Writing this book was a journey in itself. David has written many books, and discovered much as he has done so, but writing this book has probably been his greatest learning experience, for two reasons:

1. **Thinking about thinking has been a revelation**. As a philosopher, thinking, defining and theorising has been a central part of his professional life, even a place of sanctuary. At least, he felt, he had autonomy over his thoughts and ideas, even if the rest of his life was often fraught. But in reality this was a delusion.

    While not directly copied, David's ideas come from a specific, Western discipline, which he absorbed as he studied at university. All his theories, he now realises, come from that particular tradition (which is just one of hundreds of traditions of human thought). None of his ideas are original. None can be said to be his own – they come from outside, not within.

    Furthermore, to realise that he cannot control the thoughts that occur to him, and that he does not know how or why he makes most decisions, has been nothing less than a personal culture-shock: a reality check he wishes he had experienced a lot earlier in his career. Yes, he is able to decide to think about this paragraph, but where does the thought to do that come from? And why did he just sip his coffee without a thought? And why is he now gazing at a vase of flowers, thinking about the nature of colour, not this book?

2. **Ethical theories make little difference**. The tonnes and tonnes of writing and theorising about decision-making and ethics created over three thousand years of human civilisation (including his own minute contributions) are more or less irrelevant to real-life judgements. We do not make our judgements according to theories and principles; we make our judgements as human beings. We can analyse as much as we like, and we may choose to apply complex theories to problems if we wish, but we do not do this at the moment of decision-making. Something much more complex, much less certain and much less visible goes on then.

All of this has come as a shocking realisation for someone who's spent his academic life theorising and encouraging people – pretty much pointlessly as it turns out – to think accordingly.

So, we've both concluded that all of us, if we're to be realistic, need to accept that much of what we think is based on deeply, culturally ingrained myths. We list these below – six of them – and counter-balance them with what we believe to be facts.

SIX MYTHS AND SIX FACTS

MYTH ONE: NURSING AND HEALTHCARE DECISION-MAKING IS MOSTLY BLACK AND WHITE

This myth is simple to describe. It is the belief that there are rules, standards, protocols and guidelines to cover most circumstances, and that if we apply these correctly we will come up with the right answers:

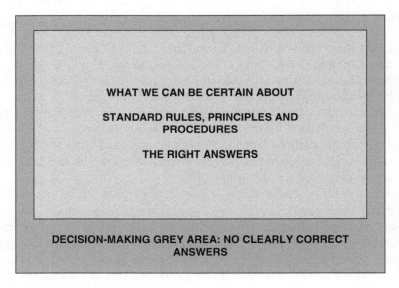

WHAT WE CAN BE CERTAIN ABOUT

STANDARD RULES, PRINCIPLES AND PROCEDURES

THE RIGHT ANSWERS

DECISION-MAKING GREY AREA: NO CLEARLY CORRECT ANSWERS

Figure 3.1   Decision-Making Status Quo

FACT ONE: NURSING AND HEALTHCARE DECISION-MAKING IS MOSTLY GREY

Chapters One and **Two** introduced several scenarios. Each can be responded to with 'fast' or 'slow' thinking. When 'slow thinking' is applied it's quickly obvious that there are no 'right answers' to be found, whatever principle, standard or rule is applied.

Recall **Scenario 1.1**, in which Mrs Suleiman, a 70-year-old widow, is recuperating from surgery to replace her hip joint, following a fall in which she fractured her neck of femur. Her son, Aashif, is insisting that she should be cared for by female staff only, according to her culture. But if you agree to Aashif's request, this would be a form of discrimination and go against the 2010 UK Equality Act, in British culture. Given this, what is the right answer?

Were **Figure 3.1** true your decision would be a piece of cake. You'd merely need to refer to a textbook, model, theory, law or ethical code, which would tell you what to do. But none of these options is actually able to do this in this case, even though it's a fairly ordinary healthcare incident. They may offer general advice, or point you in a possible direction, but they can't give you a definitive answer in these particular circumstances.

There's much less black and white and much more grey in nursing and healthcare decision-making than the myth allows. This is not only the case with ethical choices, it applies to clinical decision-making as well. Hip replacement surgery, which Mrs Suleiman has had, is also controversial and, in the end, comes down to personal judgement too. As Dr Dan Albright, an experienced orthopaedic surgeon writes:

> 'The controversy amongst surgeons is we all think that the way we do it is the best. I've done all three approaches, in my hands, the anterior approach is what I believe works the best.' **(105)**

In reality, the picture is much more like **Figure 3.2** than **Figure 3.1**:

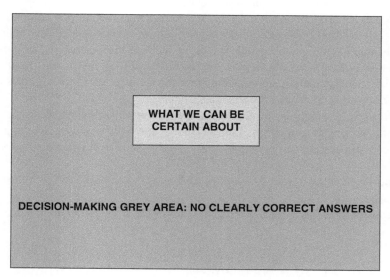

Figure 3.2   A More Realistic View of Decision-Making in Nursing

Uncertainty abounds. In the nursing literature, sources of uncertainty are said to be: unpredictable practice context; nurse–patient power balance; exposure to diverse patient needs; dealing with issues when alone; unfamiliarity with the patient and doubts about whether the patient meets the medical emergency team criteria **(106, 107)**.

The 'grey area' is not only a nursing phenomenon. It's the case for all human decision-making. With the exception of pure mathematics and associated disciplines, our thought processes must deal with constantly changing, unstable real-life circumstances, making it implausible to rely on exact algorithms and rules, even for apparently simple human decisions.

MYTH TWO: THE AUTONOMOUS INDIVIDUAL IS THE SOLE DRIVER OF DECISION-MAKING

On this myth, it's believed that our personalities, drives and values are the dominant or even the only factors in decision-making – that we make our own decisions, as individuals standing apart from everything around us: islands of decision-making, unaffected by the waters at the shore's edge.

A striking implication of this is that we expect consistency in personal judgements. If the sole driver of judgements is the individual, on the face of it there seems to be no reason to think otherwise. We're in charge, so if we decide to do X today then, in similar circumstances, we'll decide to do X tomorrow, and the day after, and onwards. If we tell the truth to a patient this week then we'll tell the truth to a similar patient next week, just because this is the sort of person we are.

A twist to this – as everybody knows – is that we supposed individual islands are not the same. I might tell the truth constantly but Sally or Johnnie might have a different drive. One health professional might be naturally candid whereas the other may be naturally reticent, and so each will make different decisions in the same circumstances. An implication of this – based on this myth – is that because we all have fixed drives and because these are naturally not the same then legislators and health officials must create regulations to make sure all individual decision-makers make the same judgements regardless of their drives, for the sake of conformity and consistency.

So, rather perversely, as a culture we revere the individual as central in society, frequently praising individualism politically, but at the same time we distrust individual judgement, and legislate to prevent decision-making diversity: the two poles of **Spectra 1** and **2**.

Of course, the biggest problem with **Myth Two** is the assumption that the legislation can actually work.

We consider this myth in more detail in **Chapter Four**.

FACT TWO: WE DO NOT STAND APART FROM THE WORLD AROUND US

The individual decision-maker is not impervious. We obviously have personalities, drives and favoured values, and clearly these affect how we make our judgements. But these are far from all that's involved in human decision-making. We're actually not islands. We are affected by the waters around us.

If we extend the **Train Journey** metaphor, the myth has us on the London tube, avoiding all eye contact, gazing into the middle distance, thinking completely private thoughts. However, numerous experiments in psychology – for example, Milgram's research on our willingness to bow to authority and Zimbardo's prisoner and guard role play (**108, 109**) – demonstrate that we're much more likely to integrate and 'group think' than we are to assert our individual values. It takes very little external pressure to change our apparently strong and permanent drives, and to radically affect our personal judgements.

We know, from the psychological literature, from our own empirical research into occupational therapists' judgements, and from half a million responses on the Values Exchange (**56**), that the individual decision-maker is not always paramount, and that we're influenced in so many ways that our expectation of consistency in individuals' judgements is misplaced. We are sometimes consistent – that is certain. But it's equally clear that sometimes with only the slightest change in ourselves or in our circumstances, we will act in contradiction to our previous choices.

We do know, as a matter of evidence, that people behave in predictable ways, according to character (a cautious, thrifty person is likely to remain that way, while a big-spender will continue to splash out). But it is also true that we're strongly affected by other people, and by our circumstances, as we explain in **Chapter Four**.

A massive body of research shows that circumstances are always a major factor in making judgements, that the individual is not actually separate from her circumstances, and that all decisions and behaviours are the result of a **combination** of the decision-maker and the circumstances.

MYTH THREE: IT'S POSSIBLE AND DESIRABLE TO OFFER HEALTHCARE IN A DETACHED, OBJECTIVE WAY

This myth is a further symptom of the separateness delusion. According to it, nurses and other health workers should be professional and courteous, but should not get personally involved. Demonstrating emotional attachment with patients is widely considered inappropriate, because it seems to blur professional boundaries. Being detached and resilient to pain and suffering is considered an asset and a strength by both health regulators and professional bodies. You're not supposed to be led by personal, emotional involvement. You're supposed to uphold professional standards, follow policy, be foreseeable, reliable, and resilient – and, above all, be consistently safe.

FACT THREE: IT'S IMPOSSIBLE TO CARE IN A FULLY DETACHED MANNER

This myth is easy enough to understand. If, as a carer, you become personally involved with patients, responding to them emotionally, there's a fear that you will offer less effective care than if you stand apart from them. And there is no doubt that this could be the case. However, the human experience does not actually permit this level of detachment. We're people and we have feelings and we cannot deny this. We can pretend not to feel. We can try to be professional and removed, but this is plainly a pretence. To decide to pretend is in itself a personal judgement.

Health carers are human beings and, therefore, cannot possibly **not** be personally involved in caring – this is a practical, logical and psychological fact. To expect them not to be is like expecting oak leaves to stay green in autumn – it's not natural. Nurses and other health carers are an intimate part of the process of healthcare. Expecting objectivity is asking for an impossible detachment. We can't detach ourselves from our experiences.

We can, of course, make measured judgements, but being involved personally and emotionally in healthcare is inevitable. It's what it is to be human. Criticising people for being people is a form of false consciousness. We need to accept and embrace our humanity, not regulate against it. Debrief, discuss, support, reflect, be self-aware, work on making better judgements – that's the vibrant human condition. Nurses and other health professionals are not members of the audience, they're participants in life's drama, and are continually affected by it, just as patients are.

It is possible to get over-involved with patients (**110**) but it's impossible not to be personally involved at all. And if you try to detach yourself emotionally this is in any case a personal decision, which shows you are already personally engaged.

Trying to numb and repress personal involvement is, in effect, to try to disengage and debilitate the essential human factor.

It's impossible to imagine dealing with the Mrs Suleiman scenario without being personally troubled by it. Any search for the objectively 'right answer' will show only that there isn't one. You have to make your own decision, at this time and in these circumstances, and you cannot do so as an automaton. You can only do this as you, with all you bring to the judgement. And whatever you decide – to continue with male carers or not – you will inevitably be challenged by others who take the opposite view. You will be aware of this, and this knowledge will also affect you, however hard you try not to care what they think and say.

There is overwhelming evidence from neuroscience and behavioural psychology (**111**) that we are both physically and mentally always part of our situations. We may not be personally ill, and may if we wish consider ourselves removed from a patient's experience, but we cannot remove ourselves from our own experiences of the situation, and this reality involves changes to our bodies (anxiety, stress, relief, laughter, spontaneous tears and so on) as well as our cognition and our emotions. Again, we're not separate observers of an objective world. We're an inextricable part of it, whether we like it or not. And given this we need to learn to cope with it, for example by using well-known techniques in 'emotional intelligence' (**112**).

MYTH FOUR: MEMBERS OF THE SAME PROFESSION SHARE AND ACT ON IDENTICAL VALUES

This is a widely held assumption. On the face of it, it appears reasonable to assume that people who work in the same profession will share the same values, beliefs and motivations, and that these will become even more similar — if not identical — with experience. As far as decision-making goes, the myth holds that because they are both members of the same profession; in similar circumstances Nurse X will make the same judgement as Nurse Y. That is, Nurse X could equally well be Nurse A or B or C because whoever she is, she will apply the same shared ethical standards and values.

FACT FOUR: MEMBERSHIP OF A PROFESSION NO MORE GUARANTEES AGREED DECISION-MAKING THAN MEMBERSHIP OF A FAMILY DOES

Expecting every nurse to think and decide like every other nurse, simply because she is a nurse, is like expecting every passenger on the **Train Journey** to see and experience the circumstances in the carriage in the same way. Or like expecting every member of a family to agree about everything (isn't the opposite more accurate?) This myth is simply a false view of the human experience and, therefore, of the nursing and healthcare experience too.

This conclusion is borne out by the occupational therapy research study we describe in the previous chapter. Our results show that occupational therapists do not have a shared set of values that they consistently apply in practice, despite the profession having a shared knowledge base and a common culture of 'enabling'. Much is open to personal interpretation. While the OT profession values 'enabling' in general, what each OT practitioner thinks will 'enable' in practice frequently differs.

Though it is true that people from the same profession usually find it easy to agree in general about the desirability of values like 'respecting' and 'enabling' clients, such value-statements provide only limited guidance to practitioners when dealing with real-world situations (113). For example, two practitioners may be committed to valuing both 'patient autonomy' and 'acting in the patient's best interests', but how they interpret these commitments may differ in individual cases. One practitioner might interpret 'valuing patient autonomy' as requiring compliance with the patient's currently expressed wishes, whatever they are, while another might regard the wishes as 'out of character' and hence not 'authentic', and so conclude that compliance with them would not be compatible with truly respecting autonomy in this instance (114). Furthermore, when the values of 'respecting autonomy' and 'acting in the patient's best interests' are perceived to conflict, which value the professional prioritises may differ both between two practitioners, and for the same practitioner in different contexts (115), as our own study shows.

A specific example of the fallacy is the present well-intentioned but misguided drive for 'values-based recruitment', where candidates for employment are required to demonstrate that they have 'appropriate values', which mostly means 'holding NHS values'. Yet 'values-based recruitment' is not possible in any consistent or even meaningful way. It's true that people have tendencies to behave according to their characters; for example, some people are more inclined to be open while others are more private. However, because decisions are an intricate and unpredictable mix of synapse and neuron responses, complex personal make-up, and unique circumstances, there's no guarantee that the same person will make the same decision in similar circumstances. Life is far too interesting and complicated for this.

In practice, this means that however much an aspiring job applicant may claim an ideal set of 'NHS values', when it comes to real-life decision-making these values – even if they are genuinely held – are only one factor in any judgement, and may have no bearing on the decision at all. Values are not always dominant in decision-making and, therefore, there's no point in trying to embed them in a profession, even if such a thing were possible.

MYTH FIVE: SINCE WE CAN AGREE AND ADHERE TO EVIDENCE-BASED STANDARDS FOR THE BEST CLINICAL CARE, IT'S EQUALLY POSSIBLE TO AGREE AND ADHERE TO STANDARDS FOR THE BEST ETHICAL DECISION-MAKING

This too is understandable. Why shouldn't there be shared standards for every part of professional practice, both science-based and the 'softer' aspects, like ethics? Surely if it's possible to stipulate best practice in one area it should be possible in all areas?

FACT FIVE: ETHICAL DECISION-MAKING IS NOT LIKE EVIDENCE-BASED PRACTICE

It's obviously important to use the evidence to ensure that the best treatments are provided in the optimum way to every patient, regardless of which health worker delivers them. But to imagine that it's equally possible to offer 'the most ethical intervention in the optimum way to every patient' is a huge fallacy.

There's no symmetry. Unlike scientific research, you can't establish 'ethical protocols' via experiment, and then generalise to all patients and all circumstances – the human experience is just not like this. Apart from well-established, evidence-based clinical procedures, there's no such thing as standardised care. All the scenarios in the book demonstrate this truth and, therefore, the need for personal judgement.

MYTH SIX: ETHICAL CODES AND POLICIES FOR PRACTICE OFFER ADEQUATE GUIDANCE TO EVERY DECISION-MAKER IN ALL CIRCUMSTANCES

This is a very common myth, across many professions, not only nursing and healthcare. All professions these days have Codes of Practice and Standards meant to guide practitioners' judgements. The Codes are often highly prized, and thought to represent the most admirable aspirations that all professionals should follow. We offer several examples from nursing throughout this text.

FACT SIX: ETHICAL CODES ALWAYS REQUIRE PERSONAL INTERPRETATION

Criticisms of these ethical declarations tend to meet a frosty reception; nevertheless, they do not and cannot do what their authors want them to. We offer many examples and explanations of this myth across the book. With the greatest respect, ethical codes don't work.

It is worth reiterating that it's one thing declaring, for example, that health carers should 'show courage and commitment' when caring for patients (13), but quite another to work out what this actually means in practice. Professionals will often disagree with one another, or disagree with patients, about which course of action is most courageous in any particular instance.

All our scenarios demonstrate that such general policy statements are always open to wide interpretation, and require personal judgement if they are to be applied meaningfully in practice.

THE MYTHICAL DECISION-MAKER

Taken together, these myths conjure up a rather strange and unreal image of a human decision-maker. This fictional creature is able to detach herself from what's going on around her, even emotionally. Her values and drives are permanent and predictable, and barely affected by her circumstances, if at all. She is willing and able to apply the best standards – clinically and ethically – to arrive at the right answers, of which in most cases there can be little doubt. Whatever happens, she will 'keep her head'. This fabulous person can even be ethical in an impersonal way, by behaving in line with ethical codes and standard policies, just as every other 'ethical person' can.

BIG ASSUMPTIONS

The six myths assume that personal judgement can and should be minimised and, ideally, eliminated from professional life. Rather than risk fluctuating, quirky choices, it's considered preferable that health carers should decide and practise according to standard evidence, values and regulations: the more sameness and predictability there is, the better the healthcare will be.

But the myths assume a consistency and level of certainty in decision-making that doesn't really exist. Such regularity is unachievable in real life, as shown by:

- Extensive research and theory in psychology which demonstrates that explicit personal choosing is just one of many factors in decision-making
- Everyday personal experience – a very simple example is that, dependent on our mood, which is in turn dependent on what's going on around us, we may make different choices in the same circumstances, for instance being rude or calm when we experience rudeness from others (this can even be affected by such simple differences as whether or not we have had coffee)
- Thousands of examples of actual decision-making – many of which are stored on the Values Exchange (**56**), which we've used over several years (we describe an example from a cohort of health professional students in **Chapter Four**). Respondents to scenarios presented by this system frequently report that they really didn't know what to think, and could have decided either way (this is borne out by their inconsistent decision-making over time when presented with similar scenarios to judge – their explicit values turn out to be just one part of a complex process of making choices)
- The results of a large empirical research project into health professionals' values which show striking inconsistencies in the professionals' judgements in commonplace circumstances (described in **Chapter Two**)
- Our own philosophical understanding of personal judgement explained in **Chapter Four**. We call this **PSP**. We believe that thoughtful reflection about the complex nature of people, about life's ceaselessly complicated events, and about the practical difficulties of arriving at complex choices consistently, also exposes the six myths.

We all make personal judgements all the time, but not in the ways the myths claim we do. We don't make aloof judgements, we make embedded judgements.

EVERYDAY DIFFICULT SCENARIOS

None of the 43 nursing and healthcare scenarios we present in this book can be adequately addressed using standard approaches alone, just as there is no regulation approach you can apply to the **Tuna Quiche** dilemma (**Chapter One**).

In any complex human situation there are always unanswered questions and choices to be made. We believe it's infinitely better to accept that 'the rules' are never enough, and that often there simply are no rules, rather than to pretend that there are authoritative protocols which guarantee the correct decisions.

We believe that while there are many different standard approaches to decision-making in nursing (some of which we outline in **Chapter Two**), without personal judgement these are never sufficient. This can be shown simply by the fact that there are different approaches at all. In any given situation some person has to decide which approach, or combination of approaches, to use. A human being has to decide: is this a legal issue? Is it an economic calculation? Is it a question of managing risk? Can the problem be solved by applying an ethical principle (and if so, which one?). Do we need to use a combination of evidence, law and ethics? Would it be best to find an official protocol to abide by? These choices are matters of personal judgement, as is so much else in life.

We offer our scenarios – most of which are drawn from direct experience – as a remedy for the misconception that we can and should limit personal judgement. We believe each scenario obviously requires personal judgement if it is to be dealt with kindly, creatively and effectively – indeed, if it is to be dealt with at all.

We assert, therefore, that sustained practice in thinking about real-world 'no right answer' examples, plus the acceptance that there are no absolute rules and procedures in cases such as these, is a must for every nurse and health carer, however novice or experienced he is. We likewise believe that practice in personal judgement applied to complex everyday problems should be mandatory for all nurse education and continuing professional development.

SUMMARY OF CHAPTER THREE

1) Human life is like a train journey. While it can be predictable – and even boring – you never know what will happen
2) No one is in a protected bubble on the train
3) Everyone can be affected by every aspect of the journey, including the physical environment of the train, the views framed by the windows, the slightest human interaction or explicit personal conflict or support
4) The mythical view of healthcare decision-making is that individuals are in charge (though we cannot always be trusted to make good decisions) and are basically aloof, detached (even reluctant) participants who can and do consistently apply uniform rules and standards
5) Compelling facts show that this 'healthcare decision-maker' is a fiction – life is much more ingrained and entwined than the myths would have us believe

CHAPTER THREE EXERCISES

Having read **Chapter Three** you may like to attempt the following exercises, to reinforce your learning:

1. Choose one of the six myths and, in your own words, write a paragraph explaining why it is false
2. Describe a decision you have made today and state, in as much detail as possible what, in your opinion, influenced you to make this decision rather than a different one
3. Describe a healthcare problem where there is no obviously right answer
4. Take a statement from your or another profession's ethical code and interpret it in two ways that could lead to different practice outcomes (116, 117, 118).

CHAPTER 4

PSP: PERSONALLY INVOLVED DECISION-MAKING

AIMS

This chapter has the following aims:

1) To describe and explain a third **Spectrum** in which the decision-maker appears separate from the circumstances and decision at one pole and an integral part of the situation at the other
2) To explain a simple theory called **PSP**, which stands for **person, situation, plan**
3) To explain an important distinction between **circumstances** and **situations** that is a fundamental part of **PSP**
4) To give examples of how exactly the same **circumstances** can be perceived by three different people to create very different **situations**
5) To explain four ways to use **PSP**
6) To explain how to use **PSP** with worked examples

LEARNING OUTCOMES

When you have read and worked through this chapter you should be able to:

1) Explain the full importance of the three **Spectra**
2) Understand the theory of **PSP**
3) Apply **PSP** to your personal life, use it to clarify healthcare situations, use it to help patients gain a deeper understanding of their situations, and use it constructively in groups to make justifiable decisions

THE POWER OF PERSONAL INVOLVEMENT

Personal involvement is the fundamental feature of meaningful human life. It's inescapable, partly mysterious, and it constantly changes our realities.

Different understandings of decision-making in nursing can be illustrated by a third spectrum (Figure 4.1) – as with **Spectra 1** and **2**, the 'hard' or more objective elements sit to the left.

We think this spectrum is actually misleading (more on this in **Chapter Eight**). We believe the left pole is not possible. In our view, it's not just nurse creativity that sits to the right, as in **Spectrum 1**, but the whole reality of the experience of being a nurse is there.

NURSE DECISION-MAKER SEPARATE FROM THE SITUATION	NURSE DECISION-MAKER AN ESSENTIAL PART OF THE SITUATION

• Nurses as observers	• Nurses involved personally in all aspects of the situation
• Nurses as objective judges	• Impossible to view situations from an objective, impartial standpoint
• Decisions and actions made from a position of detached authority	• Situations change dependent on who is involved, including the nurse

Figure 4.1   Spectrum 3

We call our idea **PSP** and explain it in this chapter. Mirroring the thoughts of many physicists that the observer is necessarily part of everything she observes (**119**), we believe that in every interaction, at every stage of her daily work, every nurse adds herself as a unique being, even when she follows protocols or uses apparently 'pure clinical judgement', and regardless of whether she performs well or badly. Because each nurse is unique, she and all that has made her what she is, mixes with the circumstances she encounters, to create one-off, unrepeatable situations.

Nursing situations do not exist apart from the nurse who participates in them: when Nurse A helps the patient she creates a different reality from that created by Nurse B when she helps the patient

To take a simple example, in Mrs Suleiman's scenario (**Scenario 1.1, Chapter One**), if the nurse involved is from the West she will create a different reality from a nurse from Mrs Suleiman's own culture simply by the way she views the circumstances: she will see a different situation from the Western nurse because of the cultural insights that are part of who she is. She will also, most likely, create a different practical reality as she works out what to do and acts on that.

It's important to try to grasp this in as much depth as possible, though we do not claim to have a perfect understanding ourselves. Knowing what **PSP** is does not mean that it becomes instantly easier to make good judgements, if anything it makes it harder at first. However, once the idea is understood and accepted, a more ingrained and imaginative form of nursing comes into view, as we explain in this book's final chapter.

PERPETUAL DECISIONS

We're apparently almost entirely powerless to affect the vast world around us. There's so much beyond our control it seems we're little more than observers, watching an epic movie someone else scripted, mere spectators of an unstoppable tide of events.

In many ways this is obviously true. In Shakespeare's ego-shattering words, we're all 'poor players' strutting and fretting hopelessly, our efforts amounting to nothing more than 'dusty death' all too soon. But seen in another light, we have amazing power. As we make and act on our judgements we influence the world in extraordinarily far-reaching ways.

Life's an endless stream of decisions. Every living action is caused by a judgement of some kind, conscious or unconscious. Should it be this way or that way? Should it be now or later? Should I do this or that? Should I make coffee or tea? Should I wear my red top or my blue one? Should I smile or be grim? Should I agree to my patient's request or not? Should I take the job offer? Should I follow norms or challenge them? Should I join with other people or should I stand apart?

It's debatable of course, but as far as we know no conscious human choice is predetermined. Rather it's up to each one of us to decide as individuals, in whatever circumstances we find ourselves.

Every choice creates a new situation and each new situation requires boundless further decisions, as new realities unfold. If you feel ill and yet nevertheless decide to go to work, your choice changes the world. The decisions you make that day affect people you would not have affected had you stayed at home, particularly as a healthcare professional. And if you decide to stay at home this changes the world too, since others' options will inevitably be altered by your absence.

We're not separate observers of an objective world. We're an inextricable part of it, connected to everything and everyone around us, past, present and future. Both in nursing and in life in general we have vastly more impact than we imagine.

We generally give little thought to daily circumstances. Life can seem so overwhelming it's easier just to get on with things. But if we take the time to contemplate even the most commonplace states of affairs, the force of personal judgement becomes plain. We do have choices. We always have choices. And as we choose we affect other beings enormously. We're not neutral objects, we're people. We bring ourselves to every situation, and as we do we change it and it changes us – just like the train journey we describe in **Chapter Three**.

PSP: THE BASIC COMPONENTS OF PERSONAL JUDGEMENT

We do not have a perfect method for good personal judgement. Nor do we have a comprehensive understanding of what it is. Like everyone else who studies human judgement, we are left with much we can only guess at.

PSP stands for **PERSON – SITUATION – PLAN**. These are its basic components.

PERSONS

As everyone knows, merely by thinking about our own lives and those of others, humans are extraordinarily complex beings.

We tend to see ourselves as autonomous individuals, but really we're connected to everything and everyone around us. In Johann Gottlieb Fichte's words:

> ... you [cannot] remove a single grain of sand from its place without thereby ... changing something throughout all parts of the immeasurable whole. (**120**)

No one's an island. We're inextricably connected to the lives of others, regardless of whether their thoughts and actions influence us directly or indirectly.

Nor are people static. We change physically, emotionally and intellectually all the time. We may wake up with no pain but stub a toe walking to the bathroom. We may wake up happy but then recall an enduring sadness. We may read a book and find our thoughts instantly affected by it. Anything can change us, at any time. Even apparently insignificant factors can make a big difference – the painful toe may stop us jogging to work, we may end up in a traffic jam instead, which might then affect our mood, leading us to make a different work decision from that which we normally would – with endless further differences flowing from that (**71**).

We're at the mercy of an incredible array of forces, almost all of which are beyond our control. We're oblivious to most of them – we make almost all of our decisions unaware of the influences that make us who we are:

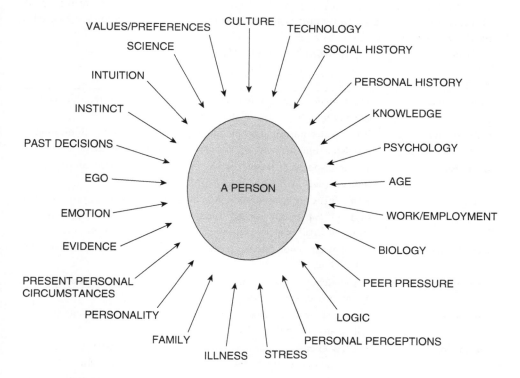

Figure 4.2   Some Influences that Create Persons

We bring these influences to every decision we make. They don't just affect us as if we are some other entity, separate from them, rather these influences **are** us.

We assume that we choose entirely rationally or logically, when in fact we're influenced by myriad unconscious factors. If we're to understand ourselves and others with any accuracy it's vital that we recognise this vast sea of forces that create us (**111, 121**).

Think about any decision you've ever made, however trivial. Did it just spring into existence? Would every other person in the world have made the same decision? It's absolutely certain they wouldn't.

Your grandmother gave you some money for Christmas. What do you do with it? Do you put it in the bank? Do you go shopping? Do you pay off a debt? Do you give it to charity? Do you refuse to accept the gift because you feel she can't afford it?

It may seem that what you decide is not worth a second thought, but if you do think about it, there are huge, hidden reasons for your choice. Say you decide to go shopping, buy some clothes maybe. That's not a neutral decision – it's not obvious. **You** made that choice to shop rather than reduce your debt. Why did you do that?

You were influenced, in some very personal way. You will likely never know exactly how – you probably won't even think about it – but you were influenced. You brought so many hidden motivations to the shops, as you bought the coolest outfit you ever owned: culture, age, emotion, ego, desire, need, peer pressure, stress, values, personal history, past decisions (failures and successes), evidence (you looked in the mirror), personality, family (will your Mum be ok with this?). You didn't just decide out of the blue. **You** decided.

You certainly did not decide objectively, that much is well known in psychology. As an individual, you were subtly and not so subtly influenced by a wide range of what psychologists call 'biases'.

There is a comprehensive list of biases here (**122**). For example:

Courtesy bias	The tendency to give an opinion that is more socially correct than one's true opinion, so as to avoid offending anyone.
Curse of knowledge	When better-informed people find it extremely difficult to think about problems from the perspective of lesser-informed people.
Declinism	The predisposition to view the past favourably (rosy retrospection) and future negatively.
Decoy effect	Preferences for either option A or B change in favor of option B when option C is presented, which is completely dominated by option B (inferior in all respects) and partially dominated by option A.
Default effect	When given a choice between several options, the tendency to favor the default one.
Denomination effect	The tendency to spend more money when it is denominated in small amounts (e.g., coins) rather than large amounts (e.g., bills).
Disposition effect	The tendency to sell an asset that has accumulated in value and resist selling an asset that has declined in value.
Distinction bias	The tendency to view two options as more dissimilar when evaluating them simultaneously than when evaluating them separately.
Dunning–Kruger effect	The tendency for unskilled individuals to overestimate their own ability and the tendency for experts to underestimate their own ability.

(123, 124)

CIRCUMSTANCES AND SITUATIONS: A CRUCIAL DISTINCTION

There's a crucial distinction between **circumstances** and **situations**. This central component of our account of personal judgement is based on a familiar phenomenon:

> **Exactly the same set of circumstances can be experienced by two different people and each may define different situations**

Commonplace examples include different people seeing sports games differently ('we deserved to win', 'no *we* deserved to win') or drawing different conclusions from the same conversations, or interpreting others' behaviours in contrasting ways, or seeing a person's character differently, or taking different meanings from the same poem.

We use this distinction to explain our view of nursing reality.

CIRCUMSTANCES

By **circumstances** we mean simple, undeniable facts – stuff that just is the case. For example, that a patient's blood pressure is 130/85, that current law says smoking tobacco in hospitals is not permitted, or that one member of staff has just instructed another member of staff to do something.

SITUATIONS

By **situation** we mean how the circumstances are perceived or interpreted by the person. **Circumstances** are what they are for anyone viewing them – in 'philosophy-speak' they're 'raw data'. But **situations** can be very different dependent on who's considering the circumstances. All the scenarios in this book can be looked at in this way. For example, here's a shortened version of **Scenario 6.1** from **Chapter Six**:

> You're working with an experienced and well-respected Health Care Assistant, Carol. You're short-staffed so you've asked her to use the staff room for her lunch break, so you can call her out if an emergency arises.
>
> You enter the staff room and are surprised to find Carol eating a hot meal from the patient food trolley. This is against hospital policy.
>
> You ask Carol why she's eating a patient's meal. She replies that she's short of money, and she forgot to bring in any provision for lunch, as she overslept this morning.

The **circumstances** simply exist, as described above. However, the **situations** are different from the **circumstances**. The circumstances 'just are' whereas a **situation** depends upon the **relationship** between the **person** viewing and the **circumstances**. For example, if you're the person viewing, you may like or dislike Carol. You may always be supportive of your staff or you may be a disciplinarian. You may be concerned about the ramifications for you personally, if you do not caution Carol or report her to a line manager. Or you may think it much more important that on a busy ward all your staff are well-fed and watered, so they can offer the best possible service to patients: two different persons, same circumstances, two different situations.

There's always only one set of **circumstances**, yet there may be many **situations**. The person making the judgement doesn't sit outside the **situation** she defines, she's part of it.

In addition, in the above example, Carol is a **person** too and will, therefore, create her own **situation** as she views the **circumstances**.

There has to be a person – to make the judgement – and there has to be some circumstances to be judged. These circumstances can be anything that exists outside the person who may judge them. The circumstances may, for example, be events (from the very largest to the very smallest) or other people's actions (from the very largest to the very smallest) or other people's characters, or works of art, or literature, or social traditions, or official policies, or news stories, or disputes between people, or conflicts between nations – the circumstances to be judged can be anything at all.

There's a two-way relationship between the person and the circumstances – the person judging colours and interprets the circumstances and, in turn, the circumstances affect the person, and are likely to affect different people differently. And, sooner or later, circumstances always change.

As Erik Hollnagel has remarked:

> People do not act on what they can see, on what is actually there and on what they have been taught. They act on what they perceive, on what they pay attention to and on what they can remember.

Hollnagel goes on to say:

> But what they perceive, what they attend to and what they remember are based on multiple and sometimes conflicting interests and motivations and are rarely if ever in agreement with the ideal of rational decisions. What people do reflects their understanding of the situation, their socially conditioned assumptions about how the world works ... as well as many other things. (**125**)

This is well known in psychology. We are simply taking matters to their logical conclusion:

> ... the same person changes his behaviour from one situation [we would say 'set of circumstances'] to another – parties, interviews etc – in keeping with different rules and conventions. People also vary their behaviour according to age, sex, and

social class of those present ... Some people behave so differently towards men and women that they seem to undergo a personality change when moving from one kind of encounter to another. **(126)**

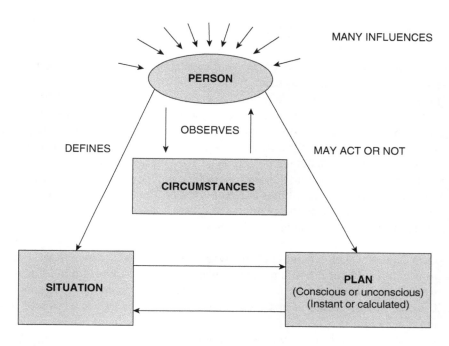

Figure 4.3   The Basic Components of Personal Judgement

PLAN

Whatever the **situation**, if you or anyone else involved wants to act – or even if you or they decide to do nothing – there will be plans. These may be trivial and disappear in an instant, if the situation is not considered important, or they may be significant and far-reaching, for example if you decide to initiate disciplinary action against Carol, who ate from the patient's meal trolley in the example above.

By 'plan' we do not mean only extensive, calculated strategies. We don't mean plans only in the grand sense of architects' blueprints or election manifestos, though these too are reactions to circumstances and situations. Rather we mean any intent to act – or not to act – whether conscious or unconscious, explicit or not. By plan we mean 'any response to circumstances', however small. For us, a 'plan' can be an instinct to flee, a nervous laugh to defuse a conflict, an unconscious choice to turn left or right on a leisurely walk, and even a bodily reaction to send white blood cells to tackle infection. All of these are personal judgements.

For the purposes of this book about nursing and healthcare decision-making we usually mean explicit plans, choices and justifications to do one thing or another, but this is not all we mean when we use the word 'plan'.

THE PHOTOGRAPHY ANALOGY

What we are saying is certainly not original, but equally it is not always easy to understand or accept. A further analogy may help.

There is a widely held and often firmly entrenched view a) that what I see in the world out there you will see too and b) that my view of the world is correct/real/true/objective/unadulterated etcetera. To show that this belief is false, think about different people taking photographs of the same scene according to a simple brief. The scene or brief can be anything at all, but for illustration let's say the brief is 'half an hour in the life of your hospital ward'. It can be the same ward for every photographer. In other words, each photographer can take whatever pictures they like of the same general, limited circumstances, during the same half hour.

Now consider the many and inevitable points of difference:

- Each camera will be different in some way. Even if each photographer were to use exactly the same model of camera there will be subtle differences in the machinery, which will affect the images. In reality, the differences in 'the human machinery' – in the photographer's senses and their ability to observe for example – will be much more marked.
- If the photographers use manual settings for their images they will choose different combinations to achieve the most effective images they can, so creating different results (warm and soft or sharp and bright, for example).
- If the photographers use automatic settings these will adjust themselves, according to the prevailing conditions, reflecting changes in camera angles and lighting which are bound to alter constantly, so also creating different results.
- The action on the ward will change continually too, making it impossible to take the same photograph twice. Photography, like human observation and interaction, happens in 'the moment', and each moment is in some way unique.
- More broadly, each photographer will interpret the brief differently and will choose different subject matter, even if only slightly different.
- Photographs have an inevitable frame, which governs what's included and excluded. Different photographers will create different frames even of the same specific scene, and will therefore include and exclude different aspects of what they see through their viewfinder. It is very common for photographers to take multiple shots of the same scene in order to choose the best version when they review what they have produced.
- The scope of the brief – i.e. what pictures are taken or not – is open to interpretation by each photographer. Some may, for example, choose to take wide angle shots of general ward activity while others may focus on specific patients, or perhaps show changing moods, using close-ups of health professionals' faces. The longer the period of time in the brief the more differences there will be.

For these reasons, even in a 30-minute period, photographers are likely to produce a wide and varied portfolio of images, to reflect their physical and emotional perspectives on the brief. Not everyone will be in a physical position to record the same events and, even if they are, they must record them from different angles. Emotionally, each photographer is likely to feel differently about the events, which will affect the images she considers of most importance. For example, dependent on whether she likes or dislikes working on the ward she is likely to offer a different version of the brief.

There isn't just one 'day in the life of the ward'. There are as many days as there are photographers.

PEOPLE ARE INCONSISTENT DECISION-MAKERS BECAUSE IT'S NOT JUST ABOUT US AS INDIVIDUALS

These quotes are instructive (**126**):

'When forming an impression of someone we tend to produce an over-simple picture of them: we assume they are highly consistent.'

'If we think about it, people are very complex, and not always consistent; the best individuals sometimes do things which are less admirable, and have their weak points, and vice versa.'

'Impressions of others are more or less subject to bias, depending on the mood of the observer. Forgas (1992) found that induction of happy or depressed moods by hypnotism or other methods has a strong effect on how people view videotapes of themselves and others.'

'An "error in personal perception" is … assuming a person will behave in the same way in other situations, overlooking situational causes of his observed behaviour, including the behaviour of the observer himself.'

'It is assumed that behaviour is mainly due to persons rather than to situations, behaviour is thought of as generated by personality traits even when it isn't … Thinking in terms of persons and their traits, rather than situations and *their* traits, maybe a pervasive feature of Western culture.'

There is a commonplace expectation that we humans are consistent decision-makers. That is, if we decide to do something, X, in a particular set of circumstances we will also do X when we encounter the same or similar circumstances. Most of us see ourselves, and others, in this light.

We like people who we see as consistent, since consistency is synonymous with being reliable and trustworthy: 'You know where you are with Billy. He keeps a straight bat. He's as good as his word.' And we tend to take pride in being consistent ourselves: 'I have consistent values. I treat people fairly. When the going gets tough I keep my integrity.'

However, even when it comes to knowledge of ourselves and others (which is after all a very personal knowledge) we are not immune from inconsistency and uncertainty. Though it may be uncomfortable to realise this, we are essentially unpredictable.

This seems counterintuitive at first sight, but then we suppose that most of this book will seem counterintuitive to many. We expect (and need) to find 'the right answers', we certainly expect to know ourselves, but even here theory and research evidence shows that while life is sometimes predictable, this is by no means always so, and human beings are no exception:

> ... the way to understand variability between situations is to analyse and take account of the situation ... not to just examine the person making them, but to examine the situation [our 'circumstances'] people find themselves in – 'personality and situations jointly affect behaviour.' (**126**).

Michael Argyle offers a simple table entitled, 'How personality and situation might affect lateness':

Minutes late for	lecture	tutorial	coffee	person means
Tom	0	3	6	3
Dick	3	6	9	6
Harry	6	9	12	9
Situation means	3	6	9	6

(**123**)

Argyle supposes that if persons and situations are equally important their lateness would make a regular pattern, and future behaviour could be predicted from this pattern. But Argyle explains:

> However ... we now know that people are not nearly as consistent as this. Harry might be keen on lectures and always arrive early, while Tom is very bored by lectures and is always late. The traditional trait model [that people's behaviour can be predicted from their personalities alone] has been replaced by an interactionist model of personality (Endler and Magnusson, 1976). This model recognises the existence of stable, underlying features of personality, but says that these interact with the properties of particular situations to produce behaviour. (p.102) (**126**)

The idea, which is in keeping with **PSP**, is that 'the influences that create persons' (our phrase) may or may not come into play, dependent on the **situation** (our circumstances):

> 'Persons high in internal control ... will stick to their beliefs and values, but do not necessarily display the same social behaviour in different situations; coping

successfully with a situation may require social moves that are specific to that situation.' (**126**)

Argyle uses the example of 'authoritarian bullies' who are more likely to bully less powerful or important people than they are to bully more powerful, dominant people. This is rather obvious, but has wide implications when seen as **PSP**.

Argyle also says:

Attempts have been made to test these two models by finding the relative importance of persons (P), situations (S) and P x S interaction. This is done by observing ... the behaviour of a number of individuals in a number of situations and calculating how much of the situation can be explained by persons and situations. The averages for a number of studies are as follows:

Persons   31.6%

Situations   21.5%

P x S   46.9%

(Furnham and Jaspers, 1983)

The overall results are very clear: persons and situations are both important, but P x S interaction is more important than either. (p. 102) (**126**)

Again, this seems obvious. For example, while Harry is inclined not to like lectures, if he has taken a fancy to a fellow student who, unlike Harry, is very keen on lectures, and gets to them early, then he is likely to arrive early too: he is the same person but one influence has outweighed another, and the **situation** (our use of the word) has changed. For us, this is the interaction between person and circumstance to create a different **situation**, and associated with that, a specific plan: get there early and sit next to him or her!

But of course it's not nearly as simple as this. In the example above we're considering only two personal influences – one trumping the other at present – and one change to the circumstances (a person Harry likes at the lecture). But the reality is exponentially more complex.

Consider this, if persons have 25 primary influences or drives, for example, each with multiple nuances and sub-drives, and circumstances have an indefinite (but clearly large) number of differences, then behaviour (or judgement) becomes mind-bogglingly impossible to predict at different times. Say there are 25 personal influences (as per our diagram in **Figure 4.2**, we are sure there are more) that might come to the fore at any one time, and 100 likely different circumstances, then the permutation of possible **situations** is simply vast (something like 10404387323078 4153964730004).

How many personal influences are in play? In what degree? How do they interact? How do they change? Do they change every minute? What are the circumstances? Who defines them? What are their boundaries for each viewer?

This seems to be a good explanation for the different – and otherwise puzzling – judgements we found in our occupational therapy values research described in **Chapter Two**. Humans and the world we interact with are just too complex and varied to be stereotyped. The bottom line is that even a highly conscientious and reliable individual may respect a client's choice in one instance and reject the choice in another, even if the circumstances seem, at least on the surface, to be highly similar.

ONE SET OF CIRCUMSTANCES, THREE SITUATIONS

To illustrate **PSP**, let's revisit Joe, whom we first met in **Chapter Two, Scenario 2.1**. Joe asked where his wife is, forgetting in his illness that she is dead.

Consider three different community health professionals judging the circumstances, which are clear and indisputable:

> *A 78 year-old-man who has been diagnosed with dementia has asked where his wife is. His wife has been dead for nearly four years, but he has forgotten. At this moment Joe believes his wife is alive.*

The three community health professionals are: **Jonathan**, 49-year-old male nurse whose father has recently been diagnosed with dementia; **Wassim**, a 27-year-old male social worker who recently completed a Master's dissertation on 'the ethics of caring for people with dementia'; and **Fatima**, a 55-year-old female doctor, Joe's GP, who's known Joe for 20 years, well before he began to be confused.

For each professional the circumstances are identical, but they are not identical people, and so each creates different situations.

Jonathan interacts with the circumstances in the following way: he feels terrible foreboding, he feels sick inside and wants to push away and deny the circumstances. It's all too much for him. When Joe asks him, 'Where's my wife?', Jonathan freezes. He hears but doesn't want to. His only thought is: this isn't my problem. He coughs, mutters something he knows Joe can't hear, looks at his watch, then rushes away.

Wassim interacts with the circumstances in a different way: he's excited but also challenged. Part of his Masters dissertation was about the ethics of truth-telling to dementia patients, mostly about telling them their condition (or not) but also about relating other factors that may affect them.

While chatting with Joe, Wassim remembers he did a 'spot survey' amongst his fellow students about a cat called Marmaduke. The issue he asked about was whether or not a person with dementia should be told that their much-loved cat – who'd been given permanently to a neighbour to look after – had been run over and killed this morning. There was little chance that the person suffering from dementia would find out unless he was told explicitly. When Joe asks Wassim directly, 'Where's my wife?' Wassim is at first taken aback and says nothing. But briefly he turns away, hiding a faint but spontaneous rueful smile – the Marmaduke survey result was exactly 50:50.

Wassim thinks quickly. In his dissertation he had argued – quite passionately in fact – that everyone has the right to know the truth, however painful that might be. But right now, seeing the fear and sadness in Joe's eyes, observing his hands shaking, it seems to Wassim that there's really no choice. Wassim feels, somehow, that even though Joe is asking where his wife is, he knows – deep down – that she's dead. He's just hoping, trapped in his muddle, that he's wrong – he's gambling on it. Today he wants to be told she's ok. He needs to be told she's ok. It seems quite obvious to Wassim at this moment.

So, Wassim takes a deep breath, holds Joe's shoulder, and says, with some presence of mind: 'Don't worry, Joe. She said she needed to go to the shops today so I expect she'll be in a little later than usual.' A flash of some emotion – shock? relief? – passes behind Joe's eyes. Then he smiles, and relaxes. 'Good. Good .... Thank you,' he says.

Fatima interacts with the circumstances in yet another way: she feels sad to see Joe like this, and she's deeply frustrated at her impotence to help him. All her studies, all her experience, all the science, all the funding – and all she can do is talk to him kindly, trying to interact as if he's still as he was when she knew him as a vital, interested editor of her local newspaper.

When Joe asks her, 'Where's my wife?' she doesn't see the illness, she sees Joe, as he was and as he is, but she sees him. And because of this she has no hesitation. 'Joe,' she says, 'I'm so sorry but Elizabeth has been dead for four years. You know deep down I think, but you forget sometimes. I know this is hard for you but I am telling you this out of respect, and so you can continue to grieve for her. I think that one day you won't ask this question any more. I'm so sorry. Shall I sit with you for a while?'

One set of circumstances, several situations, all of which emerge from the relationship between the people involved and the circumstances.

In one way this may seem a strange conclusion, if you're used to looking for **the** truth, if you think that there are ultimately right and wrong answers to all questions. Yet, given how complex and diverse people are, how could it really be otherwise?

WAYS TO USE PSP

There's a risk that what we're saying may seem hard to apply in practice. However, with practise using either scenarios or real life, it can become a very positive habit, alerting you to the complexity in even the most apparently straightforward circumstances.

PSP is not a flow chart or a systematic, step-by-step approach to problem-solving. It cannot solve problems for us. No such methods exist. But it can clarify their depth, and it can encourage careful, constructive conversations.

In general, **PSP** describes what personal judgement consists of. It shows what must be involved during any act of personal judgement. As a matter of necessity, unless there is a person and something to be judged there can be no personal judgement. And once there is a decision – conscious or unconscious – then a plan exists. This three-way relationship between persons, situations and plans reflects a constantly changing, dynamic environment, quite unlike the flow-chart approaches we considered in **Chapter One**.

GENERAL PSP — AND A SIMPLE TEMPLATE

In its most general form, **PSP** can assist in understanding your own and other people's decision-making in all circumstances where there's uncertainty about what should be decided. It cannot, of course, decide for you — that is a matter of personal judgement.

This is how to apply **PSP** in general. Say to yourself, in these circumstances there are people involved, there are situations that are defined differently by different people, and there are, therefore, different plans. Ask:

Person

- What people are involved? What influences does each bring with them? What are their goals at this moment?

Situation

- How do you frame and scope the situation? How do you think others frame and scope the situation?
- What factors are most important to this situation? What factors can you exclude?

Plan/Means

- What approach/approaches will you use to make your judgement? What approach/approaches will others use? How specifically will you decide?

In order to support personal judgement specifically, in practice, and to offer concrete ways for nurses and other health workers to work in such fluid realities, we suggest four different ways to practice with, and to use, **PSP**. These may be applied to any of the scenarios in **Chapter Five**.

The four versions are:

PERSONAL PSP

For personal use in life – as a way of promoting self-awareness and insight into your own way of judging.

Personal **PSP** suggests that you need to observe the influences that make you who you are (as in **Figure 4.2** above). It encourages you to work out how these influences interact with prevailing circumstances to create the situation you see.

Ask: what influences me? How do I define the situation to be judged? Why did I define this situation rather than a different one? What problems do I see? Are there problems that I have overlooked? When I personally decide what to do, how do I do that – how do I weigh and balance the situation?

HEALTH CARER PSP

PSP can be used by you as a health carer, as a way of promoting insight into your way of making judgements as a health professional.

> **Ask: what influences me in my professional practice? Do I define the situation to be judged or do others do it for me? Are the problems I see the same as others see? How do I decide what to do – is there a difference between what I am expected to do as a professional and what I feel I should do personally? If so, how do I feel about this? How do I go about resolving these differences?**

This version of **PSP** might also be used in situations where accountability is important. It can help you, in a rounded, personal way, explain and justify your decision-making to others, where this is required. You can say how you – as a unique person – created the situation, as you saw it. Rather than saying 'I followed the nursing process' or 'method Y' you can say, 'I brought myself into this situation – this is how I thought and felt and this is how I saw it.'

This is an honest way to be, and since there are no absolute rights and wrongs in caring situations, this should build confidence in your reasoning ability. This is not to say that all ways of solving problems are equal – there are practical and philosophical reasons why they are not – but it is to say that your genuine personal attempt to understand and to intervene is valid.

PSP FOR USE WITH CLIENTS/PATIENTS

PSP can be used as a very simple method for clarifying patients' priorities, in keeping with contemporary interest in 'person-centred decision-making'.

> **Ask the patient: what situation do we need to deal with? What are the main problems? What worries you most?**

> **Explain to the patient: this is the situation I believe we need to deal with. These are the problems I see. These are the priorities as I see them. I make these judgements as a human being, trying to be as aware as possible of what influences me as a person.**

When there are two **PSPs**, which is very often the case when professionals and patients are tackling a particular set of circumstances, the key task for both parties is to explain their **situations** as clearly as possible to each other.

PSP FOR USE IN HEALTH PROFESSIONAL GROUPS

PSP is a way to explore social realities with groups of people.

One way to use **PSP** to broaden and deepen understanding is to have different people in a group each create their own personal PSP template – and then compare them together, so as to generate rich discussion and, ideally, come up with a practical solution to the problem at hand.

Method: Each professional member of the group should first use PSP personally. Ask: what influences me? How do I define the situation to be judged? What problems do I see? How do I personally decide what to do?

Then, as a group exercise, each member might explain her personal **PSP**, and then consider, 'Do I define the situation to be judged or do others do it for me?' 'Are the problems I see the same as others see?' 'How do I decide what to do – is there a difference between what I am expected to do as a professional and what I feel I should do personally?'

This option is particularly useful in debriefing.

APPLYING PSP TO THE WOMAN AND THE DOG

In **Chapter One, Scenario 1.3,** we considered a recurring situation where a 60-year-old woman repeatedly calls an ambulance to take her to A&E, complaining of acute, severe abdominal pain. However, on arrival her pain quickly subsides. We learnt that she brings her dog into the department and can therefore skip queues – since the dog has to be kept outside for health and safety reasons – and she gets all the attention and care she demands (including hot drinks, food and blankets for her, and a bowl of water for the dog) because she has to wait with her pet. This continuing pattern upsets both patients and staff, and there is disagreement over what to do about it.

We applied various approaches to nurse decision-making to this case and found them to be of little practical use. Does **PSP** fare any better?

There are many alternative judgement supports, and we do not say that **PSP** is ideal or the best method, but we do think it is worth including as part of your decision-making equipment.

Applying **PSP** to the case of the woman and the dog explicitly brings out the personal, and allows us to view the issue richly, from a range of possible personal perspectives – rather than say assigning points to a range of possible outcomes, and applying these according to some formula or other.

Using **GENERAL PSP** we can ask:

PERSON

What people are involved? What influences does each bring with them? What are their goals at this moment?

Straightaway it can be seen that personal judgement is immediately required to answer even the opening question. Even deciding which people are involved requires reflection, a decision and, ideally, an awareness of what factors caused you to decide who to include. For example, are the people temporarily in the A&E department on this day involved with the general issue (whatever you decide that is), given that they will probably only experience it once? Are the ambulance staff involved, after all they merely deliver the woman to the department, as is their duty? Is the Head of Department, who's never actually met the woman, involved? There seems to be no way to decide this objectively, and it seems equally clear that different decision-makers might well see things differently.

It helps if a clear question, or proposal about what should be done is put forward, but of course this too is personal. For example, there is quite a difference between 'I propose that the woman is banned from the Department' and 'I propose that we set up a multidisciplinary team to support the woman and get to the bottom of this problem'.

Once you have decided who is involved then you have to work out how they are influenced, which may not be possible for several reasons, and what their goals are, which might be achieved by asking them. And if these goals are different then – somehow – if you have the power at all, you need to work out which are most important.

While this level of uncertainty may seem troubling – very possibly disorienting – it could be easy enough to make a decision, you just need to be aware that it's impossible to assess objectively whether or not it's the 'right' one.

SITUATION

How do you frame and scope the situation? How do you think others frame and scope the situation?

What factors are most important to this situation? What factors can you exclude?

This is the biggest question – what you see as the **situation** is likely not to be the way others involved see it. Indeed, different people may take the same circumstances – a woman repeatedly visiting A&E and achieving no resolution – and create very different realities. It may be that the locum doctor today sees the **scope** of the situation narrowly – just a matter of working out how best to proceed on this day – whereas the triage nurse sees the scope over an extended period, stretching to the future, and quite possibly involving other patients too. And it may be that the woman patient frames the situation as unwillingness of the hospital and its staff to help her, whereas the triage nurse frames the situation as a selfish, needy person manipulating everyone to boost her ego.

The different people involved quite literally create different mental realities, as they perceive what is happening, and as they act they create different physical realities too. There is no objective situation.

This may seem disempowering – how on earth can I make a sensible decision when so much is so variable? – but it is ultimately more enabling than disabling. If you take a fixed view of a fluid reality you are unlikely to arrive at the most effective ways to help. But if – instead – you try to take a respectful view of the different realities, you can intervene thoughtfully and creatively, and humbly. You can, for instance, talk to all involved, ask them how each sees the situation, and then lay out these different realities to give insight to all concerned. You might – openly and honestly – say to the woman that some staff think she is malingering, and ask her to respond to that. And you might say to the staff that the woman feels scared, abandoned and confused about what is wrong with her.

There are many other options that might break the deadlock, but the important thing is to find some path, some way forward, that will change the circumstances and therefore make different situations (interpretations, realities) possible: a shift is needed. This requires the ability to see things from others' perspectives, the willingness to be flexible, the ability to translate people's views of the situations to others, and ideally to have a guiding purpose you are committed to following as a health worker, and that you can share with and explain to others (we believe this purpose should be to create as much autonomy as possible).

MEANS/PLAN — AND PSP PLUS

What approach/approaches will you use to make your judgement? What approach/ approaches will others use? How specifically will you decide?

We described ten possible approaches in **Chapter Two.** One or more of these can be used in combination with **PSP** – we call this **PSP PLUS**.

PSP PLUS — FOR USE IN HEALTH PROFESSIONAL GROUPS — APPLIED TO THE WOMAN AND THE DOG

Let's try a different form of **PSP PLUS** other approaches, and imaginatively consider an informal team meeting using it.

———— SCENARIO 1.3 REVISITED WITH ————
PSP PLUS

THE TEAM MEETING

SCENE: HOSPITAL CANTEEN

Characters: Jessica, Simon, Adam (an ambulance driver), Sanjeev (a doctor)

Jessica and Simon are eating lunch at a table in the canteen. Adam and Sanjeev walk over with trays and ask to join them.

Simon: Sure guys, very welcome.

Adam and Sanjeev take seats opposite Jessica and Simon.

Sanjeev:	Just salad today?
(*to Jessica*)	
Jessica:	Obviously Sanjeev. What of it?
Sanjeev:	Woah, sorry. It was just a light comment.
Jessica:	Are you saying I'm fat?

Sanjeev and Adam look at each other, a little perplexed.

Simon:	Well if anyone should be on a diet it's me (he leans back and pats his rather
(laughing)	large belly, with a satisfied grin).
Jessica:	Actually I'm not on a diet. I am going vegan for the month. It's Veganuary. I'm sure you've heard of it?

The others look blank.

| **Jessica:** | It's an idea that started a couple of years back, to encourage people to stop eating animals. Actually, to stop using any animal products at all. It's healthier all round. |
| **Sanjeev:** | I'd like to see the evidence for that. What about protein? |

Jessica gives Sanjeev a despairing look. Adam quickly changes the subject.

Adam:	Talking of animal rights, what are we going to do about *that* woman and *that* dog?
Jessica:	You know what I think already. She's a total time-waster. She should be barred from the hospital. She takes up everyone's time when we have real emergencies going on around us all the time. I'd call the RSPCA about the way she treats the dog too.
Simon:	We've been through this a few times. It's not kind, we don't know what's
(*firmly*)	wrong with her, and in law we have a duty of care to her. I know it is frustrating but we do have a duty, on many levels.
Jessica:	We have a duty of care to everyone that comes in here. She takes resources from the others. We have a duty to get rid of her. Let her GP have the pleasure of sorting her out.
Sanjeev:	What's this about?
(who works elsewhere in the hospital)	

Jessica briefly explains that the woman attends every few weeks complaining of severe abdominal pain, which vanishes as soon as she is seen and assessed by the team. She demands attention and must have special support outside the department's building because of her dog. Simon nods.

| **Sanjeev:** | Is there nothing physical? |

(Continued)

Simon:	We can't find anything, not ever. But we have to bring her in because she presents with severe acute abdo pain, despite a lack of objective signs.
Sanjeev:	Have you referred her?
Simon:	To who? Anyway, she leaves as soon as we've seen her. She gets angry. Says we're no use, that we just don't see her properly, because she's old and will die soon anyway. She basically storms out when we tell her we don't know what's wrong.
Adam: *(to everyone)*	Next time she calls, if I'm on duty, should I just refuse to bring her here do you think?
Sanjeev:	That might be risky to you, if there really is something wrong with her. What's her name by the way?
Jessica:	Daisy. Daisy Greenwood. You know, if you do bring her in then we should refuse to treat her. Tell her to go back home and see her GP.
Simon:	Don't you think we're legally bound to assess her at least?
Jessica:	We're legally and ethically bound to act in the best interests of all our patients, and potential patients. Not just one.
Simon:	Are we? I'm not 100% clear on the law here. I think we need to check.
Sanjeev: *(who's been fiddling with his phone)*	Where does she live?
Jessica:	She is in our catchment area but other than that I don't know. I don't care really.
Simon:	That's harsh, you know.
Jessica:	Maybe it is. (*She shakes her head negatively*) I've just had a gutful of time wasters to be honest and her yappy dog drives me wild. She smells pretty bad too. She looks like she hasn't had a bath for months!
Adam:	I know where she lives because we collect her. She lives very locally. Dorchester Avenue. On her own, I think. Apart from the dog.
Simon:	What's her dog called? Do we even know that?
Adam:	I do. I have to tie him up in the ambulance for safety reasons. He doesn't like it so we have to calm him. He's called Yorkie. Daisy and Yorkie, the dreadful duo we call them.
Sanjeev:	Is this her?

Sanjeev holds up a picture of a woman in an old newspaper article, on his phone.

Jessica:	(*at a quick glance*) Could be I suppose. If it is, she's lost loads of weight since that photo.

Simon: May I see?

Simon looks at the picture and then reads the article. The headline is **SINGLE MOTHER IN LEGAL BATTLE WITH LOCAL HOSPITAL: alleged negligence in sudden death of 11 year old.** *There is an accompanying picture of a* **Daisy Greenwood, local resident,** *standing outside the doors of the A&E Department, as it was in the 1990s. The article describes how Daisy's son – Jason – presented to the A&E Department with acute abdominal pain, was sent away due to a lack of objective signs, and later collapsed at home with a perforated appendix. Jason died in hospital a short time afterwards from peritonitis and shock.*

Simon passes the phone to Jessica.

Simon: It must be her mustn't it?

Jessica: It's not certain.

Everyone looks shocked, humbled and uncertain of what to say. Eventually Sanjeev speaks.

Sanjeev: This is a really tragic story. I wonder if Daisy has ever received any therapy for the loss of her son?

Even Jessica seems reflective now. She starts to refer to 'that woman' as Daisy. They all agree that maybe Yorkie provides vital companionship for Daisy, after a bereavement that many would find difficult or impossible to recover from.

Sanjeev: Next time I think I would call the liaison psychiatrist, or the whole team should maybe try and talk to her about the loss of her son. And maybe a referral to bereavement therapy? Does everyone agree?

Jessica: Would it help though?

Sanjeev: Well, I think because she presents with the same symptoms and the same conclusion is always reached, then this is very triggering for her. We have to bear in mind that her son was also sent away from here without the team finding objective signs, and without any help, all those years ago. This could explain her behaviour – maybe she's just looking for someone to blame still, or maybe she's challenging us to do better. Or perhaps she's still trying to make sense of what exactly happened to Jason. Or maybe somehow her behaving like this makes Jason still real – even still alive – for her?

I wonder if she ever received an admission of liability from the hospital? Or compensation? It would be incredibly hard for her if she didn't receive that closure, or didn't even receive an explanation that she could live with ... wouldn't it?

They all sit in silence, reflecting on the story of Daisy and Yorkie.

HOW IS PSP DIFFERENT FROM STANDARD NURSING MODELS?

We do not recommend **PSP** as a method or a pathway to follow – rather it's merely a short-hand illustration of how we see the **content** of personal judgement. And it is with this content – the stuff of judgement – that we are most concerned. We want to enhance personal judgement in nursing, and that means enhancing the understanding that there is never just one reality that everyone sees the same, there are always many realities to negotiate.

That said, it's fair to say that in some ways what we are saying is standard – identify the problem, work out what to do, and do it effectively. It's hard to disagree with such pragmatism. However, we're seeking to inform pragmatism with a very different view of what's really involved in human decision-making, as follows:

1. Typical nursing decision-making approaches (though not all of them) assume an objective view of a set of circumstances that are seen in the same way by everyone – and that there is a right answer to be found (and often an approved approach). By contrast, we believe everything is personal, fluid and in flux. There are no impersonal decisions.
2. We do not think of reflection as a stepwise, linear process. Rather it's liquid and dynamic, is often all tangled up, and cannot be adequately described or prescribed in flow charts and the like (even though these devices can be useful in a limited way).
3. We believe that reality – including nursing reality – changes according to who's observing and who's involved. The reality of daily practice is not fixed. The nurses involved affect reality.
4. We emphasise the processes rather than the outcomes. We want everyone to real-ise how personal the process of making judgements – any judgements – in health-care actually is.

THE DIFFERENCE BETWEEN EMPATHY AND PSP

None of this is to say that it is easy, or even fully possible, to 'step into someone else's shoes'. It is not uncommon to hear 'empathy' cited as a positive value, and also to hear that to care well for another person it's important to be 'empathetic'. But in fact 'empathy' is a difficult notion, both conceptually and practically.

At its simplest, the idea is that if you can feel another person's pain and distress in some way, then this will make you kinder. Research does indeed show that if another person's experience becomes salient to you then this is likely to happen, but there are significant problems with empathy, including:

*   It's much easier to empathise with people who are like ourselves. In fact, recent research shows that taking the perspective of someone who has opposite or conflicting attitudes actually make you less empathetic, because this forces you to think in a way that is incongruent with your own values, and diminishes your receptiveness (**127**)

- Empathy exhibits favouritism, as neuroscience has shown. Brain areas that correspond to the experience of empathy are sensitive to whether someone is a friend or a foe, part of one's group or part of an opposing group. And they are sensitive to whether the person is pleasing to look at or not, and much else
- We may not understand the other person – we may empathise with our version of what the other person is feeling rather than what she is actually feeling. The fact that we very readily project our own thoughts, emotions and biases on others is something health carers must constantly bear in mind: am I empathically listening to what another person is needing and feeling or am I hearing only how it would be for me if I were in the other person's shoes? How can I be sure that my feelings of empathy are entirely and accurately towards another person rather than my imaginary view of them?
- Apparently, empathy can even spark violence: our feelings for the sufferer can motivate anger towards whoever caused the suffering. According to the *Guardian*, this idea was summarised by Adam Smith in 1759:

> When we see one man oppressed or injured by another, the sympathy which we feel with the distress of the sufferer seems to serve only to animate our fellow-feeling with his resentment against the offender. We are rejoiced to see him attack his adversary in his turn and are eager and ready to assist him.

> There is now laboratory evidence for such a relationship – which shows that people who are highly empathetic tend to be more violent and punitive when they see someone who is suffering. (**128**)

For these reasons, it is important to be clear that **PSP** is not just a different way of empathising and nor are we recommending that health professionals should be empathetic. Rather we are emphasising the complexity of understanding ourselves and others, the power and unpredictability of the many forces that drive us, and the need to be constantly aware that the way you see a situation is almost certainly in some way different from the way others see it, and is very possibly radically different.

What we are saying is that however much you feel you may have empathised with another person you can do this only as **you** – and this may well mean that your feeling that you have fully understood another person – or another person's situation – may be illusory. We can strive for empathy if we wish but it may always escape us, and we should be aware of this, while finding as many ways as possible to allow other people to express themselves, as themselves.

SITUATIONS AND CIRCUMSTANCES – A SIMPLE HEALTHCARE EXAMPLE

Here is a simple scenario that was presented to students, via the Values Exchange, as part of their Interprofessional Education at the University of Derby, in the UK.

Students were asked to consider a brief scenario, and then decide whose needs are the most important. How they chose indicates how they define the **situation**.

—— SCENARIO 4.1: A FAMILY IN CRISIS ——

CATEGORIES: RESOURCES, PRIORITISING, FAMILY

Dad, Stuart, is not coping as a newly single parent bringing up his teenage son, Rob, and pregnant teenage daughter, Tilly. He's not looking after himself properly and appears to be drinking heavily.

Son, Rob, is not coping well with his Mum's death and has stopped talking. He has just sustained a head injury after falling off his bike, 20 minutes ago.

Teenage daughter, Tilly, is pregnant. She may have mild learning difficulties and is struggling to cope with being pregnant, and to understand what is happening to her. She met the father online. He is no longer around.

Source: Tim Howell, the University of Derby

As a group this is how they responded on the Values Exchange (20/11/18):

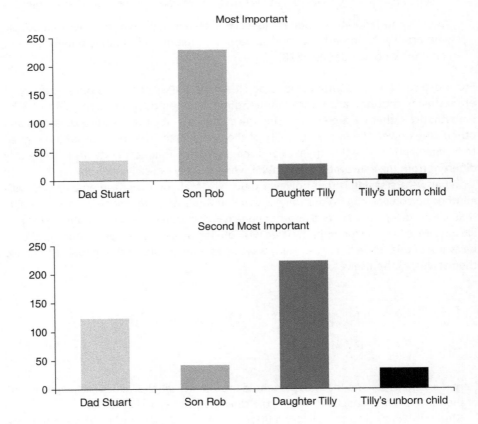

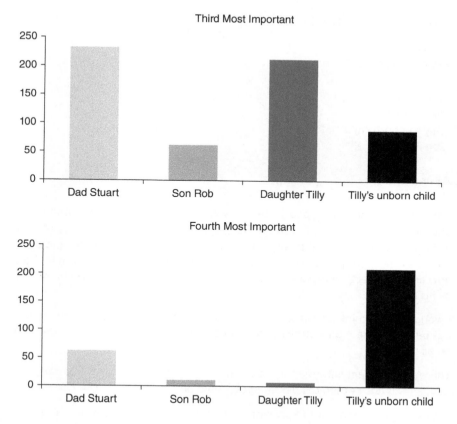

Figure 4.4   Scenario 4.1 Poll Results

If you think son Rob's needs are most important then – according to **PSP** – you're picturing a different situation from someone who thinks Tilly's needs are most important.

We did not picture the same situation ourselves.

USING PSP WITH TILLY

PSP makes us aware, first, that we are all unique persons, influenced and formed by very many factors; second, that it is each one of us, personally, who defines situations; and third, that if we want to bring about change then we, personally, have to make or adopt a plan that we can justify.

DAVID'S PSP: WHAT INFLUENCES ME?

David's ranking order:

1. Dad Stuart
2. Daughter Tilly
3. Tilly's unborn child
4. Son Rob

David's rationale:

I think that if Dad gets support then he will be able to support the others, and this will greatly help his self-esteem. To me he seems most vulnerable, not least because as a man he is culturally expected to be strong – to 'man up' and cope. But he's clearly struggling. I can see major mental health problems for him, both now and, I suspect, increasingly as more and more demands are placed upon him by his children.

I wonder if I'm thinking this because I too am a father who has had trauma and has been expected to be strong and to cope? I do empathise with Dad, I think (as far as I can).

There's insufficient information about the son's head injury. I'm assuming it's minor, for if it isn't then the paramedics should be called to action.

I think Tilly is second most important because she is second most vulnerable.

Looking at **Figure 4.2** I am drawn to the following influences, in particular:

• PERSONAL HISTORY

• PERSONAL PERCEPTIONS

• PAST DECISIONS

• LOGIC

I am aware that these shape who I am at this moment, and I feel, though cannot prove, that these are the most powerful factors informing my ranking order, and also the most important factors as I decide what to do.

HOW DO I DEFINE THE SITUATION TO BE JUDGED?

I see the situation as a complex family dynamic, in which communication is very poor. I see Dad Stuart at the centre of everything. He has no wife to help him and he does not know how to talk to his children, nor do they know how to talk to him, but they both need his support very much.

I understand that others see the circumstances differently, and so create different **situations**. The results of the survey tell me that most respondents – who are healthcare students – put Son Rob at the centre, or at the pinnacle of concern, because of a possible serious head injury. Yet this is not my focus, this is not the situation as I see it. Even if Rob does have a serious injury he needs the support of his father, and his father needs to respond as the head of the family.

WHAT PROBLEMS DO I SEE?

The inability to communicate well. A family under great stress, facing a kind of defeat. They have lost Mum and now they face permanent disintegration as a family.

HOW DO I PERSONALLY DECIDE WHAT TO DO?

Were I a nurse with some power to intervene in this situation I would do my utmost to relax Dad and have a supportive conversation with him, looking at a range of practical options he could pursue both for himself and his offspring.

VANESSA'S PSP: WHAT INFLUENCES ME?

Vanessa's ranking order:

1. Son Rob
2. Dad Stuart
3. Daughter Tilly
4. Tilly's unborn child

Vanessa's rationale:

Rob needs urgent medical assessment and bereavement support.

Stuart also needs bereavement and alcohol dependence help as soon as possible, so that he can care for himself and therefore support his teenage children.

Tilly needs routine support throughout her pregnancy but has a little time on her hands to work through her difficulties (not sure what her current gestation is?).

Tilly's unborn child is safe as long as Tilly receives proper antenatal care throughout her pregnancy.

I am influenced by my previous clinical training, especially where a head injury is concerned.

I am also influenced by my father who struggled taking care of my brothers, who were teenagers, when my mother left and divorced him. He coped by increasing his alcohol consumption to survive with his 'bereavement'. He became lost in his own problems and my brothers became hard to support and manage as a result.

I am influenced as a mother too. I know that Tilly has a gestation of 9 months and will receive automatic support from antenatal services and the GP at least, as long as she is able to interact and access these supports.

I am influenced by my personal and professional knowledge of knowing that if Tilly is cared for by her father and professionals collaboratively, then Baby will be fine in utero, until she is delivered at least. And Tilly can be enabled and educated to allow her to take on more individual self-care throughout her pregnancy, and support her family unit in doing so also.

HOW DO I DEFINE THE SITUATION TO BE JUDGED?

I define the situation as a family who are struggling to cope with the devastating death of their mother, and as a result, the children are engaging in risky behaviours (maybe as a cry for attention to their needs). The father is lost in his own world of grief, drinking heavily and thus struggling to support his children. They're all expressing their grief in non-therapeutic ways, resulting in dysfunction and although they are physically together, they are emotionally isolated from each other.

WHAT PROBLEMS DO I SEE?

- A potentially serious head injury
- Individual and collective grief
- Lack of motivation and helplessness
- Risky behaviours
- Communication breakdown
- Lack of support and understanding
- Future family fragmentation if not addressed

HOW DO I PERSONALLY DECIDE WHAT TO DO?

By listening to my perception, and applying my experience, my knowledge and my intuitive insight into this situation.

I would ensure that the son was out of imminent physical danger from his head injury as a priority, with thorough assessment and follow up. I would then offer some crisis counselling to dad and 'signpost' him to alcohol dependence services (with consent). This should empower him to become more self-aware and to gain the strength needed to support and supervise his offspring. I would also organise family therapy for them collectively (if they are willing) and ensure that Tilly has access, opportunity and reasonable adjustments to carry through her pregnancy. It's important to help her understand and make choices on behalf of her own care provision, and the future care of her unborn child.

I don't see any benefit in referring to social services, as this may further fragment and disengage the family, unless imminent danger to the children is apparent. I think they need understanding in the context of their situation (which has come about through no fault of their own) and extensive bereavement support. A referral to an OT may also be beneficial to enable the family to function in a practical way which benefits all collectively and individually.

SUMMARY OF CHAPTER FOUR

1) Personal involvement is the fundamental feature of meaningful human life. It's inescapable, partly mysterious, and it constantly changes our realities
2) We're at the mercy of an incredible array of forces, almost all of which are beyond our control. We're oblivious to most of them – we make almost all of our decisions unaware of the influences that make us who we are
3) We assume that we choose entirely rationally or logically, when in fact we're influenced by myriad unconscious factors
4) Nursing situations do not exist apart from the nurse who participates in them. When Nurse A helps the patient she creates a different reality from that created by Nurse B when she helps the patient
5) There's a crucial distinction between **circumstances** and **situations**. Exactly the same set of circumstances can be experienced by two different people and each may define different situations
6) There's a two-way relationship between the person and the circumstances – the person judging colours and interprets the circumstances and, in turn, the circumstances affect the person, and are likely to affect different people differently
7) Consequently, we propose a new approach to nurse decision-making, which we call **PSP**
8) **PSP** stands for PERSON – SITUATION – PLAN
9) We offer a simple **PSP** template and suggest four different ways it can be applied in context
10) We also suggest **PSP PLUS** – in which **PSP** is combined with one or more of ten classic decision-making approaches in nursing
11) We illustrate **PSP** with the examples of Joe who suffers from dementia and who has forgotten that his wife is dead, Daisy and Yorkie who regularly disrupt A&E, and a dysfunctional family seen differently through the eyes of different students

CHAPTER FOUR EXERCISES

Having read **Chapter Four** you may like to attempt the following exercises, to reinforce your learning:

1. Create a new **Spectrum** that incorporates the three **spectra** introduced in this book
2. Explain the difference, as defined in this chapter, between **circumstances** and **situations**
3. Describe **PSP** in your own words
4. Explain **PSP PLUS** and say why it is useful for healthcare decision-making
5. Apply **PSP PLUS** to your choice of scenarios in **Chapter Five**
6. Apply **PSP** or **PSP PLUS** to a challenging set of circumstances you have experienced in your personal life

CHAPTER 5

PRACTICE SCENARIO:
AN EXEMPLAR

AIMS

This chapter has the following aims:

1) To offer an exemplar scenario that is more fully worked through than other scenarios
2) To place the **PSP** template conveniently in this chapter for easy access

LEARNING OUTCOMES

When you have read and worked through this chapter you should be able to:

1) Apply the **PSP** template in your own way to Bill's scenario
2) Better understand the importance of scoping and framing in personal judgement

We spend more time looking at Bill's case than any other scenario in this book. We do so because we consider Bill a particularly good example of how different people see the same circumstances and create vastly different situations from them.

SCENARIO 5.1: CONDITIONAL COMPASSION?

CATEGORIES: PATIENT CHOICE, STAFF CONFLICT

Bill, a 78-year-old man, was widowed six months ago. Bill is in the post-op recovery stage following a total hip replacement three days ago. Apart from some mild Atrial Fibrillation, Arthritis and Reactive Depression (since the sudden death of his wife, Edith) Bill is considered to be reasonably fit and well. No complications for discharge are anticipated.

As an experienced return to practice (**RTP**) nurse on the unit, you've noticed that Bill appears to be more withdrawn since his operation and frequently keeps his door shut. Today you knock and enter. You find Bill sitting in his chair, beside his bed, shuffling cards on the table in front of him. As the ward is quiet, you ask if he would like to partner you in a few games of Pontoon. Bill smiles weakly, accepts and gestures for you pull up the chair opposite him.

While playing, Bill starts to talk of how he played cards every day with his wife. Suddenly his eyes fill up and he begins to cry. You move the table away from in front of him and move from your chair. In an attempt to get closer and adjacent to Bill, you sit on the bed next to his chair and hold his outstretched hand.

A few moments later, the Staff Nurse walks past the door, which is still ajar. She raises her voice and tells you to 'get off the bed, it's against policy'.

In order to prevent cross infection it is Trust Infection Control Policy for staff to refrain from sitting on patients' beds. But due to lack of space the bed is the only way to sit next to rather than opposite Bill, as there is no room to move the chair by his side.

On hearing the Staff Nurse's command Bill looks worried and alarmed. He tells you, 'you should go, I don't want you to get into trouble on my account.'

What do you think you should do? Do you agree with the proposal below?

EXAMPLE PROPOSAL FOR FOCUS: It is proposed that you ignore the Staff Nurse and remain seated on the bed in order to comfort Bill.

Note: a version of this scenario first appeared in *Thoughtful Healthcare* (**69**)

THREE DIFFERENT SITUATIONS

The circumstances are as described above. However, there are at least three very different **situations**. These are experienced by the:

- Return to Practice Nurse
- Senior Nurse
- Bill, the patient

THE RTP NURSE'S SITUATION

I am a return to practice nurse on the Unit. I've been caring for Bill (under supervision) since his admission. I've noticed that he appears to be more detached since his operation and frequently keeps his door shut.

I feel I have developed a real connection with Bill since he's been on the ward. I recently lost my own grandmother to cancer, and the empathy I feel for Bill, at this difficult time, has been enhanced by reflecting upon the difficulties my own grandfather has struggled with. The ward is reasonably busy but I'm a supernumerary staff member at present, therefore I take advantage of my status, on this particular day.

I put on a disposable apron, wash my hands, knock and enter. I find Bill sitting in his chair beside his bed, shuffling cards on the table in front of him. Bill looks pleased to see me. I ask if he would like to partner me in a few games of Pontoon. Bill smiles and accepts. He gestures for me pull up the chair opposite him.

While playing, Bill starts to talk of how he always played cards with his wife. He begins to cry. I feel a need to be responsive to Bill – I move the table away from in front of him and move from my chair. In an attempt to get closer to Bill I sit on the bed next to his chair and hold his outstretched hand, which he offers to me gladly. My actions feel like a natural and appropriate reaction to Bill's distress. I know that sitting on the bed is against hospital policy, due to infection control and risk, something the unit has taken very seriously since infection outbreaks a few years ago. However, I consider that Bill is low risk – his wound is covered and intact, there's no port of entry, and his immediate need for supportive intervention is of more importance to both myself and I think to him, at this moment. This is intuitive to me. Besides, the only other place to sit, due to lack of space, is in the chair opposite and further away from Bill, as there's no room to move the chair adjacent to him, which would be the ideal place. I feel that to use the chair to sit opposite him would be inappropriate and not conducive to this therapeutic intervention, which involves touch.

I briefly consider getting up to close the door, but I feel this could break the 'caring responsiveness', in which I am currently engaged, so I stay where I am, even though I'm conscious of people walking by outside the room.

Then the Staff Nurse – our link for infection control – walks past the door. She deliberately raises her voice, ordering me to 'get off the bed'. She says I 'should come and help out on the ward'. Immediately I feel embarrassed, guilty, humiliated, anxious and angry with the senior nurse.

Bill looks worried and tells me I should go. He doesn't want me to 'get into trouble'. I feel concerned for Bill. I feel that if I get up the moment will be lost, and I feel concerned that he may not feel comfortable in future if I engage with him, in case he feels it would get me or even someone else into 'hot water' with this nurse. I naturally don't want to get into trouble with the nurse, as she is my mentor and assessor, and the senior nurse in charge, but I feel very strongly that she was wrong to do this in front of Bill, and that she has overestimated any infection risk to him. I have become increasingly aware of late of the need to demonstrate compassion. I'm also under the impression that the senior nurse is very rule driven, especially concerning the need to reduce infection risk. I always use universal precautions such as frequent handwashing and wearing a clean apron with every patient. I feel the senior nurse has not seen the big picture here and has reacted without thinking this through properly.

I decide to ignore her and remain seated on the bed for five more minutes in order to reassure Bill and comfort him. I prepare to challenge the Staff Nurse once I leave Bill's room, which is scary to me but necessary I feel. I think it's in Bill's best interests.

I hope it doesn't affect my assessment ...

THE SENIOR NURSE'S SITUATION

I am a senior nurse. I've worked on the unit for the last six years. I'm also the current lead for infection control on the unit. I'm in charge of the unit on this late shift.

We're one trained nurse down and the ward is busy with patients coming back and forth from theatre. I've just had a row with one of the doctors who changed the order of the theatre list without communicating this to anyone on the unit.

I reluctantly decided to delegate the care of Bill to the **RTP** nurse, Natalie, under supervision. Natalie is very compassionate and has been caring for Bill over the last few days when she's been on shift. Continuity of care is important to me, however I do feel concerned that Natalie has been getting a little too close to Bill. She spends a lot of her time attending to his needs behind his closed door – sometimes, I feel, to the exclusion of others.

Natalie has three other patients to care for on the unit. I feel she needs to be more aware of time management and appreciate that she can't just spend 20 minutes in Bill's room whenever she's passing the door. Even though she does have supernumerary status, she needs to work as part of a team and help out with other patients, like everyone else. I do sometimes feel that it would be nice to spend all this time sitting and talking to patients myself. But there are tasks that need to be done and I'm constrained by the responsibilities of my role.

Natalie needs to learn to prioritise better, and focus on fundamental skills like those laid out by the intentional rounding initiative, which is in place on the unit. Nurses should spend about five minutes with each patient every hour, responding to care prompts, which are written on a chart checklist. These intentional rounding charts are measurable and audited, so it's obviously important that they're adhered to.

I've just returned from an infection control update. I'm keenly aware of the need to keep staff and relatives off patients' beds, and to enforce proper handwashing and universal infection control. We don't want another **MRSA** outbreak like the one we had a couple of years ago, which closed the unit for a while. Matron is also a stickler for infection control and regularly pops onto the ward to check.

When I passed Bill's room I felt naturally cross that Natalie had the audacity to sit on the bed. After all, she's well aware of policy and I expect her to adhere to it, like everyone else. I couldn't believe she'd put Bill at risk like that. And then to top it all, she ignored me and didn't come out for another five minutes.

I am worried that Bill will become too dependent on Natalie and may even become unwilling to go home when he's discharged.

BILL'S SITUATION

Bill's sitting in his chair, beside his bed, alone in his hospital room. Through the window he can see a row of Lombardy poplar trees bending in the wind, defining the road toward the hospital gates. And beyond them, the concrete towers, chimneys, spires and domes of the awkward, messy city he's known all his life. Bill looks up once in a while, but mostly keeps his head down. All he wants to see are the shiny playing cards he's idly shuffling.

There's a knock on the door. Natalie, a **RTP** nurse walks in, smiling. She's observant and naturally thoughtful. She sits opposite Bill and asks spontaneously:

'Would you like to play cards for a while? The ward's quiet right now.'

It's the first time she's seen him smile. She thinks even a wounded smile is better than no smile, so she accepts his gesture to sit opposite and they begin to play pontoon. She laughingly suggests he ought to be banker as 'the senior partner' and they agree to play for the matches she uses to light her break-time cigarettes.

'Twist' she says, and from nowhere a vague memory of a dance-hall 60 years away floats into Bill's mind. He looks up. He sees Edith, 17, beaming, impossibly beautiful, ridiculously happy. With a jolt, Bill realises Natalie's holding his hand. He realises he's crying.

'I loved her all my life. We were together for 59 years. I don't know what to do any more ....'

The moment is shattered by a shrill command.

'Get off the bed nurse. It's against policy.'

The bossy voice immediately moves on to other rooms, leaving Bill and Natalie shocked and uncertain. Defiantly, Natalie stays on the bed.

'Please, you'd better go or you'll be in worse trouble.'

With that Bill picks up the cards, returning to his shuffling.

'It's not your fault. She's obsessed with the rules, that's all. I can play one more hand if you like?'

Bill replies hesitantly. 'Ok, but just one.'

After a minute or two Natalie gets off the bed, reassuring Bill.

'OK, I'll drop by later to see how you are.'

Rattled, confused and a little angry, Natalie walks to the door. Bill stares bleakly after her. He gets up to close the door in case anyone else tries to talk to him. He moves to the window, resting his hands on the sill, gazing down on the city, their city, their past. He looks blankly at his hands, an old man's hands, hands that are less and less to do with him, some other person's hands.

He turns and opens the drawer of his side table. He picks up a brown leather-bound book. Two photos of Edith fall to the floor. He gently places them on his card table and begins to write.

TUESDAY. AUGUST 27TH.

Dearest Edith,

Today I thought I saw you. It was only for a moment but it was real to me. We were at the Palais de Danse. I think it was our first date.

I know everything comes to an end. I know you can't read what I write to you. I know you're not here anymore. I know it but I won't accept it.

There was a kind young nurse today who tried to cheer me up, but now I feel even worse. All kindness has gone, Edith.

Bill closes the book then climbs into bed. Turning to one side he stares silently at the tilted trees. (**129**, **130**, **131**, **132**)

APPLYING PSP

USING THE GENERAL TEMPLATE

In this case, **GENERAL PSP** and the **Template** might be applied with reasonable success, to reflect on this scenario:

PERSON

- What people are involved? What influences does each bring with them? What are their goals at this moment?

SITUATION

- How do you frame and scope the situation? How do you think others frame and scope the situation?
- What factors are most important to this situation? What factors can you exclude?

MEANS/PLAN

- What approach(es) will you use to make your judgement? What approach(es) will others use? How specifically will you decide?

PERSON

What people are involved? What influences does each bring with them? What are their goals at this moment?

There are three people directly involved, this much is certain. Others may be involved indirectly, but it is not clear who, so we can limit our perusal to three people: Bill, Natalie and the Staff Nurse.

The way the scenario is presented has granted us a privileged insight into some of the influences on each person; there's more guesswork in real life. Even so, we cannot be sure if we understand all the main influences, or how much each one influences the person proportionately, but we do have a general idea.

And their goals are clear too, or at least this is how it appears – they're just not compatible.

SITUATION

How do you frame and scope the situation? How do you think others frame and scope the situation?

What factors are most important to this situation? What factors can you exclude?

It depends who 'you' are. You can be 'you' the reader, or imagine you are one of the three participants in the drama, or you can imagine you are some other person: Bill's daughter, the CEO of the hospital, a visiting ethics lecturer, Natalie's father. Whichever you choose in your imagination, he or she will see a different situation. The task for someone, somehow, is to try to understand the different perspectives in such a way as to offer a way to get the most positive way forward.

What factors are most important? What can you exclude? It's a question of judgement – you can say that 'infection control' is of paramount importance, the decisive factor, as the Staff Nurse believes. Or you can say, with Natalie, that infection control is a minor consideration, or entirely irrelevant, compared to the need to comfort Bill as a human being in need.

Natalie already decided to sit on the bed; the question now, if you want to ask it, is how should Bill be cared for tomorrow? Should Natalie still be his nurse? Should she be allowed to sit on the bed? Should she be disciplined? What should happen next?

MEANS/PLAN

What approach(es) will you use to make your judgement? What approach(es) will others use? How specifically will you decide?

One way to look at this question might be to insist that hospital policy is adhered to. Another might be to assess the likely consequences, somehow balancing costs and risks against likely benefits, as we see in some of the approaches in **Chapter Two**. And another might be to assert a legal and ethical duty to care for Bill as he wants to be cared for.

Once again, which you choose may depend on many factors, but will ultimately be a personal preference.

WHAT WOULD YOU DO NEXT, AND WHY?

You can find various models and approaches outlined in **Chapters One** and **Two**. You may also find the ideas and methods explained in **Chapter Eight** helpful. But whatever way of judging you think works best, be absolutely aware that the primary decision-maker is you.

CHAPTER FIVE EXERCISE

Apply your own version of **PSP** to Bill's scenario.

CHAPTER 6

PRACTICE SCENARIOS: STAFF AND PROFESSIONAL ISSUES

AIMS

Chapters **Six** and **Seven** have the following aims:

1) To offer realistic scenarios from many areas of nursing and healthcare
2) To encourage readers to reflect on the scenarios in order to become more aware of the astonishing real-life complexities involved in even apparently mundane circumstances
3) To encourage readers to reflect on the scenarios in order to become more aware of their personal reactions to and reasoning about these scenarios
4) To encourage readers to become more aware of how **situations** are created personally as they consider the scenarios
5) To offer further practice with the **PSP** template
6) To make optional suggestions about which decision-making approach(es) to use after each scenario

LEARNING OUTCOMES

When you have read and worked through these chapters you should be able to:

1) Propose justifiable and sustainable solutions to real-life problems in nursing and healthcare
2) Better appreciate how your personal characteristics affect your interpretation of circumstances
3) Be more aware of the depth and extent of your immediate 'fast thinking' reactions to circumstances
4) Gain experience in 'slow thinking' deliberation about your immediate reactions and be able to offer in-depth, reasoned justifications for your final opinions
5) Be able to apply the **GENERAL PSP** template as you deem appropriate

INTRODUCTION

Each scenario in the next two chapters has no right answer and might be resolved in multiple ways. Ultimately, whatever conclusion you arrive at about each will be a matter of personal judgement.

Each scenario offers proposals for consideration. We do not necessarily agree with these, they are there to provide focus only. We do give our own reflections on each though we do not claim to be right. While there are facts that we try to clarify, our personal reflections are simply how we see matters at this point in time, as the people we are at present.

The best way to improve personal judgement is to practise, to exercise your reflective powers in challenging circumstances, where different facts and perspectives compete. We offer these scenarios in this spirit – for deliberation, to enhance self-awareness, and for discussion with others.

ORGANISING THE SCENARIOS

Because we present numerous scenarios, we've divided them into three **chapters**: the exemplar scenario in **Chapter Five**; in **Chapter Six,** we offer scenarios that focus on staff relationships and conflicts (the area of practice where personal judgement is often most needed and most challenging); and in **Chapter Seven,** we present scenarios that impact most directly on patients and families. Admittedly, to divide up the scenarios in this way has an arbitrary element since all the scenarios involve both staff and patients. However, we hope that placing the scenarios like so makes them easier to digest and use.

— SCENARIO 6.1: MAKING A MEAL OF IT? —

CATEGORIES: STAFF BEHAVIOUR, RESOURCES

It's a very busy day in your department. You're working with an experienced and well-respected Health Care Assistant, Carol. Staffing is at a minimum and there is not enough staff to allow each to leave the ward at break times for a 30-minute, uninterrupted break. Instead, you've asked Carol to use the staff room for her lunch break, so that you can call her out if an emergency arises.

It's lunchtime on the unit. After the patient meals have been given out, the trolley is pushed to the exit of the ward, next to the staff room.

Ten minutes later, you enter the staff room to use the toilet. You're surprised to find your colleague eating a hot meal from the patient food trolley, which is clearly against hospital policy.

You ask Carol why she's eating this patient meal. She replies that she's short of money and forgot to bring any provision in for lunchtime as she overslept that morning and only just made it to work in time.

What would you do in this situation? Do you agree with the proposal?

EXAMPLE PROPOSAL FOR FOCUS: It is proposed that you report Carol to the unit manager for eating patient food off the trolley.

VANESSA'S REFLECTIONS ON THIS SCENARIO

I would not report this, if it were a one-off incident. Instead I would have a chat with the member of staff, to see if there is anything I could help with. I would also say that she needs to ask in future, and not just take food from the trolley (even though it would probably be thrown away, as it was surplus) since this could be seen as professional dishonesty and is theft, a legal offence, and not something to be taken lightly. This is also a serious disciplinary offence from an employer's point of view, and can result in instant dismissal if theft, regardless of context.

However, I think we've all been in this situation, where we don't have enough cash on us or haven't had the time to make sandwiches due to other pressures. I personally think staff should have a free hot meal while at work, especially if they can't be released from the ward for a break, due to lack of organisational resources – this just seems like common sense to me, if we want to retain staff and keep them motivated. The organisation has a legal duty to take care of staff and provide adequate break provisions. However, I don't think that the meal should come from the patients' food trolley – and if it does, it has to be because no patient requires it first.

I think there's too much eagerness to report people when this type of issue arises – and we need to be more understanding and compassionate, and consider the context. I would rather be looked after by a member of staff who has had a decent meal than one who hasn't. However, if this were happening routinely then I would raise a concern, as it could get out of hand. I have seen instances where staff have earmarked meals for themselves before they have been given out to patients, and this is obviously wrong on all counts. I have even witnessed nurses eating meals in the bathroom, when they can't be released for a break, so that they won't be overlooked by others.

What I am certain about is that we do need to look after our NHS workforce properly, by providing the resources to allow them to leave the ward, with others ideally, for a break, and so that they can talk and debrief with each other informally over a meal. We also need to ensure, if we are not able to release people from the ward for breaks that they have sufficient food and fluids to enable them to work optimally.

DAVID'S REFLECTIONS ON THIS SCENARIO

Perhaps because I am neither a health professional nor a natural rule follower, I cannot see too much to be concerned about in this situation. I can see that it could be regarded as theft and that other staff and patients could be upset by the flagrant disregard for policy, but I don't really see the point of the policy. If the food would otherwise be thrown away, and if the nurse is hungry, and if it will improve her concentration when she gets back on the ward, then to eat the meal seems a positive option: more pros than cons.

I can definitely imagine the contrary view, and I can think of people who would not only stop Carol and tell her off, but actually report her for breaking policy and the law, but it does not seem humane to me. To report her would surely be deliberately to seek to cause her harm, and it is not easy to justify causing unnecessary harm to other people.

So I would not report her. I would briefly discuss the issue and tell her what I think and I would suggest that if she needs to take food from the trolley in future she does it more discreetly, and that it would be best that it doesn't become a habit. But that's all. That would be my personal judgement in this case.

SUGGESTION FOR SCENARIO 6.1: APPLY PSP TO THIS SCENARIO PLUS THE NMC CODE

SCENARIO 6.2: THE BED MANAGER AND THE DUTY OF CARE

CATEGORIES: STAFF BEHAVIOUR, RESOURCES

You are the Senior Nurse in charge of a busy, short-stay 18-bed surgical ward. You currently have 16 patients on the ward awaiting surgery or recovering from very recent surgery. You have 2 staff nurses who've been allocated 8 patients each. One staff nurse is off sick.

During the busy shift, the bed manager for the NHS Trust that employs you rings to say they wish to transfer another patient, Paul Smith, onto your ward. Mr Smith is recovering from a fractured neck of femur following a recent fall at home, and underwent surgery to repair the fracture the day before. He's considered to be moderately dependent at present and has not commenced mobilisation therapy as yet.

You inform the bed manager that you currently have a staff nurse off sick. You have no extra capacity since the nurse-to-patient ratio is already at the nationally recommended limit of 1:8. You also explain that the patients you have already are in need of a high level of care due to their degree of dependency.

There is no other nursing assistance available to you, due to high sickness levels throughout the hospital. Although you do have two spare beds, and you would like to take care of this patient, you feel you don't have the resources to do so safely, without placing your existing patients and staff at risk of harm.

(Continued)

On hearing your position, the bed manager becomes hostile, refuses to accept your explanation and informs you that since you have an empty bed the patient must be transferred over to you anyway, as there is simply no room on the other wards, due to patients waiting to be transferred from Accident and Emergency department.

What should you do? Do you agree with the proposal below?

EXAMPLE PROPOSAL FOR FOCUS: It is proposed that you stand your ground and refuse to accept the patient.

VANESSA'S REFLECTIONS ON THIS SCENARIO

Standing up to this kind of daily pressure and coercion is easier said than done and there can be covert or overt ramifications for those who do. That said, the ramifications – legally, professionally and ethically – could potentially be worse for a nurse who continues to accept patients when she knows resources are insufficient.

The gentleman waiting to be admitted will no doubt be anxious to get to a ward to receive specialist care, which is totally understandable, and morally I would want to care for him. However, there are also currently 4-hour targets in emergency departments, which means that ideally patients should be admitted or discharged within this time scale or the Trust will be penalised. These ideals, and sometimes unreachable and unrealistic targets, place a lot of pressure on unit managers and bed managers alike. And I'm sure that the bed manager in this case is also very much under pressure from her superiors and senior clinicians to manage the situation at hand.

However, there is no legal duty of care to someone who is not proximal to you, they need to be close enough to you for your actions or omissions to affect them (this is known as the neighbour principle). However, there is a vicarious duty of care on the Trust, but not on you as a professional individual unless the patient arrives on the ward and you greet them, which would establish a legal duty of care on you.

I have witnessed this type of situation many times, where bed managers ignore a Senior Nurse's concerns about accepting a patient, and they are sent over anyway, without agreement. This is always detrimental to all involved, no matter how much we would wish to care for these patients in an ideal world.

This kind of pressure from bed managers can result in further staff shortages if those nurses under pressure fall ill and go off sick with long-term stress as a consequence. In my opinion, this shows why nurses must develop the knowledge and courage to defend their justifications and be resilient and assertive – developing the strength to make and justify their own judgements.

Most of all though, I feel passionately that nurses put in this position need support and leadership from their line managers, under their employment duty of care. Rather than having to cope repeatedly with stressful fire-fighting, the employer should provide the opportunity and time to talk about these issues in a mature way, in open dialogue, on a frequent basis. These discussions, wherever possible, should also involve the bed managers, so that everyone can appreciate each other's own pressures, and a higher level of respect can arise from these debriefing opportunities.

In this scenario, I would assure the manager that currently Mr Smith is being cared for in A&E, hopefully under close supervision, which is something I could not offer at present. I would convey that I would continue to assess patients who may be able to be discharged early with support or transferred to other areas (again not ideal for those being moved around). However I would continue to decline to accept the patient under current conditions. I would calmly explain that if the situation changes I would reassess and inform the bed manager as appropriate. I would also personally document my concerns and justifications, for the record.

DAVID'S REFLECTIONS ON THIS SCENARIO

This issue is interesting because with more information, which I would have in the real world, it would be helpful to apply **PSP**. Having said this, I am becoming increasingly aware that whatever technique one uses to analyse problems, it is artificial, at least when deciding 'in the moment'. One's human, personal reaction is much more influential than analysis. But at least **PSP** does help to show this.

The suggested way to think about this issue (below) is to use **PSP** plus the law, though you could use **PSP** plus any of the other approaches just as well. I would probably choose to use **PSP** plus the Ethical Grid if I were to carry out a full analysis, since the Grid includes the law alongside 19 other factors that may be pertinent; however, for this reflection I am most interested in **PSP** on its own.

As far as the law is concerned in this case, I am not an expert. I would – if I were often in this situation – do some research or contact legal advisers so I could be better informed and prepared. I do know that the hospital has a legal duty to offer an acceptable level of care to Mr Smith, so somehow or other the hospital must provide a bed and meet his health needs, wherever this bed is found.

In this case – applying **PSP** – the following persons are directly involved: the senior nurse, the bed manager and Mr Smith. Others – other staff and other patients – might also be involved, but I will consider only the three main protagonists, for brevity.

(Continued)

It seems to me – thinking about the senior nurse's and Vanessa's reaction – that it is easiest to imagine how they create the **situation** they see. There is a strong sense of being bullied, possibly a sense of territory (this is MY ward). Certainly, there is a sense that the ward is more important than the hospital in general – and there is antagonism toward the bed manager, and vice versa. So, I ask myself, how does the situation appear to the bed manager? I don't know and can't tell from the information in front of me but I assume the bed manager is also under pressure, has targets to meet, and may also be stressed in his or her job. Is he or she 'hostile' or 'frustrated', or something else? How does she see the problem?

Whatever the bed manager's situation, it would make sense for him or her to try to appreciate the nurse's situation, and she to do likewise for the bed manager. Do they need to be challenging each other or could they work together? They both wish to support Mr Smith, so could they work on a shared strategy and approach the hospital authorities in an alliance?

At the same time it's also important to try to conceive of the patient's situation (how does he perceive the circumstances?). Mr Smith will most likely be anxious and unsure. This is not a normal situation for him, though it is for the health service staff. While there is a dispute between the staff, and he has no place to go, his health is likely to suffer (whether physical, mental or thought of as his autonomy).

While I accept that I have no direct experience in this area, and may therefore be envisaging an entirely false situation, I disagree with Vanessa's choice on this occasion. I would accept Mr Smith onto the ward and arrange a meeting with the bed manager to look at **PSP** together and, if possible, to come up with a plan to take to the health authority to try to bring about positive change.

SUGGESTION FOR SCENARIO 6.2: APPLY PSP TO THIS SCENARIO PLUS THE LAW AND OR THE ETHICAL GRID

SCENARIO 6.3: SHOULD I STAY OR SHOULD I GO?

CATEGORIES: STAFF BEHAVIOUR, RESOURCES

You are a health professional working with a busy community team, which offers a 24-hour service to patients.

The team is experiencing a very busy Saturday, with four new acute cases to assess and continuing high dependency caseloads. The team is struggling with skeleton staff, due to high sickness levels.

You're on an early shift. Although it's been a very busy day, with no break so far, you're looking forward to attending your best friend's son's birthday party this afternoon, after you finish your shift. Her boy, Jack, is best friends with your 6-year-old son, Ben.

An hour before the start of the late shift, a nurse, who's due to work the next shift, rings in sick, saying she's started vomiting. The professional in charge informs the team manager on call, who states that there is no other help available to cover this sickness, and insists that you stay on to do a 'double' shift.

You explain you've other family commitments that afternoon, and although you frequently do cover sickness at short notice, you have noticed a decline in your health lately and you are therefore reluctant to agree this time, stating that you need to take better care of yourself to avoid stress-related sickness. Also you know that your best friend, as well as Jack and Ben, will be bitterly disappointed if you don't attend the party, where you were expecting to help with food and other preparations.

The team leader begs you to stay and explains that without your help the community team will be at unsafe staff-to-patient ratios.

What would you do in this situation? Do you agree with the proposal below?

EXAMPLE PROPOSAL FOR FOCUS: It is proposed that you leave the team at the end of the shift and attend your best friend's son's birthday party.

VANESSA'S REFLECTIONS ON THIS SCENARIO

This scenario is a common issue, which has come up frequently in my past clinical experience, and I'm sure resonates with many.

I'd feel several emotions. I'd feel worried – for my team, for the pressure they're under, and for the patients for a likely reduction in the standard of care they'll receive. I'd also feel worried for my friend, who's relying on me to be there for her, for a significant event.

I'd feel pulled from both sides. I'd feel like I couldn't do right for doing wrong.

I'd also feel upset and annoyed that I'm being pressured and coerced by the Senior Nurse to stay, because I'd feel I'm not being given proper freedom to choose. I'd also feel devalued for not having my health concerns listened to. There's always a danger of long-term sickness when we don't look after ourselves and always say 'yes' to requests of this kind. There has to be a balance between work and play, duty and self-care, if we

(Continued)

wish staff to remain resilient and able to carry out their vast and complex responsibilities to patients and staff.

I would need to ask myself, am I being exploited?

On the surface, it looks like if you say 'yes' then you're putting the patients' and the team's best interests first, but long term, are we actually? When a lot of people are off sick it's a 'red flag' sign – things can quickly turn very unsafe very quickly when staff–patient ratios are not able to be met.

Exercising my various spheres of accountability, I think my **plan** would be to:

a) Reassert my concerns to the senior nurse, apologise, but continue to state that I am feeling unwell and it would not be in the long-term best interests of either the team or patients (or my family and friends) to stay. I would also state that since I do not feel well it is unfair to pressure me.

I would be willing to offer a compromise and maybe come back to do a few more hours after an hour or so at the party, which would help release other team members to implement fundamental care. Or I would stay for a couple of hours until someone else is found to take over – if I thought it would help and I could manage this realistically. However, when we don't expose gaps, and senior management don't see what is really going on, this can be counterproductive – an exercise which veils the real issues which are occurring, resulting in the team not getting the extra resources they need. No different from 'shooting oneself in the foot', so to speak.

b) Since this is a recurring issue, I would also put this in writing to my team manager (so I could leave an evidential trail of me accepting my limitations, my concerns over this issue for my team and patients and how I felt pressured by the senior nurse on duty, even though I understand and can relate to her reasons for this).

c) I would explain my reasoning for not staying, focusing on the long-term ramifications which could come from this situation if I had decided to stay (risk, health and well-being and eventual potential lower staffing levels, leading to detrimental care, possible liability for myself, team members and the Trust vicariously, and possible disciplinary and professional misconduct issues which may arise from negligent care). I would also state the perceived benefits of my decision not to stay.

d) More long term, in taking a leadership role for my team, I would attach clauses from the **NMC Code** which I thought this action would be in breach of, clauses from my employment contract of duties, and I would also quote laws and statutes which I feel the current levels of staffing undermines.

e) I would request a reply in writing and ask for a team meeting to address this issue, so that plans could be put in place to address stress and its management, sickness and retention issues, and interventions to address and maintain patient safety and individualised care.

DAVID'S REFLECTIONS ON THIS SCENARIO

I can understand how difficult this situation would be for a sensitive, dutiful, caring health professional. In many ways it would be much easier if the professional saw her role merely as a job of work, a means to the end of making money only.

Seen this way, this case illustrates the importance of **PSP**, or some form of it. To the 'sensitive carer' the circumstances will look very different from the way they appear to the 'it's just a job' health professional – two very different situations will be seen.

If I were a nurse I would feel similarly to Vanessa – I wouldn't want to put patients in jeopardy but neither would I want to let my friend, and the two boys, down. I think that how I would decide would depend upon my own personal circumstances and feelings at the time – this is entirely in keeping with **PSP**, where the same person can make conflicting choices in very similar circumstances – as circumstances and people change then so do situations. If I were feeling particularly keen on my work, or particularly attached to my colleagues and the current set of patients, then I would be more inclined to agree – if I were feeling aggrieved and alienated for some reason, then I might instantly decline.

I don't think there is a generally right answer here. It could go either way. But what is most important is that I am self-aware, that I perceive my variability and the influences on me, and that I can on reflection consider whether my decision was justifiable, and also think carefully about what I will do if and when it happens again.

SUGGESTION FOR SCENARIO 6.3: APPLY PSP TO THIS SCENARIO PLUS THE FOUR PRINCIPLES AND YOUR INTUITION

SCENARIO 6.4: RESPECT WHERE RESPECT IS DUE?

CATEGORIES: NURSE/DOCTOR CONFLICT, LAW, CLINICAL EXPERTISE, RIGHTS

You are a seasoned nurse, with many years' experience, currently working on a medium-stay elective surgical unit.

You are on the morning shift, looking after a woman named Diane (47), who is currently in the theatre department undergoing a Laparoscopic Cholecystectomy (keyhole removal of the gallbladder) under general anaesthetic. It's intended that Diane will be cared for on

(Continued)

the unit as a day case. It's expected that she will have an uneventful recovery, allowing her to be discharged by 8pm.

Diane has a history of prescription drug dependence, which she attributes to generalised osteoarthritis, a delay in the diagnosis of her gallstones (which presented as recurring back pain) and to the length of time she had to wait for surgery (6 months). Diane says her dependence on codeine is all in the past, following a successful programme of Cognitive Behavioural Therapy (**CBT**). This information is clearly laid out in the referral letter from the GP to the Anaesthetist and Surgeon performing the operation.

At noon you receive a phone call at the nurse's station from the recovery team to say Diane is ready to come back to the unit. You are asked to fetch her.

During recovery handover you notice Diane has been prescribed Paracetamol Oral for pain relief and an anti-emetic for the post-operative period. You immediately feel, from experience, that this pain relief will not be adequate for Diane's post-operative needs. You're aware that patients recovering from this type of surgery often experience different levels and types of pain (abdominal, visceral, parietal and shoulder). From experience, you're also aware that despite the wide use of intra-abdominal local anaesthetic infiltration into wound sites with local anaesthetic during procedures, some patients often suffer from moderate to severe pain in the hours before discharge. If their pain is not managed well some patients end up in an overnight bed.

Normally, the anaesthetists prescribe either Paracetamol in conjunction with a non-steroidal anti-inflammatory drug (**NSAID**) or an opiate, dependent on individual medical history, consultant preference and contraindications. However, on this occasion neither of these analgesics has been prescribed.

When you look at Diane in the recovery room, you notice she's wearing an oxygen mask and – from her non-verbal language – appears to be in discomfort, grimacing and holding on to her stomach. You approach her and ask her to score her pain from 1 to 10 – she says it's a 6. You ask the recovery nurse why Diane hasn't been prescribed anything stronger than Paracetamol. The nurse tells you the anaesthetist will be out in a moment and to ask her directly. She also assures you that Diane has received optimum pain relief (IV) and local anaesthetic infiltration into her wound area during the procedure, and has also received Paracetamol suppositories (1g) in recovery, 30 minutes previously. You notice that Diane reported her pain as moderate to severe (pain score 8) 35 minutes ago, before she was given the Paracetamol.

The unit is getting ready to close for the day, as there is no afternoon list scheduled and the nurse excuses herself to get on with her chores. Once the morning staff leave (including the surgeon and anaesthetist) it's routine for the on-call houseman to take over the surgical care of the morning patients.

You wait to speak to the consultant anaesthetist, who has a reputation for being unapproachable and irritable. Eventually she appears. You approach her and explain that Diane appears to be in moderate to severe pain still. You ask if she can prescribe Diane something a little stronger than Paracetamol. She responds rather abruptly. She says Diane has received adequate medication during surgery so she won't be writing up anything further for her. The anaesthetist then briskly states that she is going home.

You insist that Diane is clearly still in pain and, in your experience, patients undergoing this procedure need a lot of pain relief in the post-op period. You suggest that if she could just write something else up, you'll be able to give it quickly to Diane, should she need it.

The doctor becomes aggressive. She says, 'You're a nurse, I'm the doctor. I was there during the operation and I can assure you that she doesn't need anything else written up.' Then she tells you she's going to complain to your manager about your attitude.

You take Diane back to the ward and immediately ring the on-call surgical houseman to write up the medication for Diane. You wait 30 minutes for the doctor to arrive, who then wants to examine Diane. The doctor writes up the stronger medication after examining Diane, and remarks that she doesn't understand why Diane was only prescribed Paracetamol in the immediate post-operative period.

Diane has to wait a total of 90 minutes to receive her medication, at which point the pain becomes hard to manage. Diane receives regular and strong medication throughout the night. She's eventually discharged from the unit after 48 hours of recovery.

What should you do? Do you agree with the proposal below?

EXAMPLE PROPOSAL FOR FOCUS: It is proposed that you report the incident to the anaesthetist's line manager.

VANESSA'S REFLECTIONS ON THIS SCENARIO

I would report this either to my own line manager or the anaesthetist's manager. In my opinion the doctor in question was negligent to Diane and contributed to her having to experience a protracted level of pain and an extended stay in hospital, at the expense of both the NHS and Diane and her family who were expecting her home after a relatively short stay.

The doctor owed Diane a professional standard of care, which I feel has been unreasonably breached in this instance. She failed to write up adequate pain relief (which might have been due to Diane's addiction issues in the past). The suffering caused was foreseeable and the result of the doctor's omissions.

I feel that the doctor let her personal feelings of being challenged by a nurse cloud her professional judgement and as a result this incident became a battle of wills. No one should be in pain when it could be managed, including those who have suffered addiction issues in the past.

This scenario actually happened to me while I was in active practice. I felt very angry about the outcome and the effects on Diane. It seemed a clear injustice to me while it was occurring. I recall reporting this to my manager, who was equally upset by the doctor's behaviour and attitude. However, because this doctor was known to have a bad temper, the manager did nothing about it as far as I am aware, and no feedback came back my way either.

(Continued)

This was disappointing but it's not unusual in clinical practice if others feel intimidated by those who are regarded as senior on the hierarchy. I did document this incident in the clinical notes, recording that Diane suffered a delay in receiving adequate pain relief. I also made a personal record/statement of the incident in a factual way, which was free from personal opinion, which could have been used should I have been called to account for my own actions or omissions within this scenario.

DAVID'S REFLECTIONS ON THIS SCENARIO

Our suggestion below is to try to use **PSP** plus the 'four principles', as an experiment, to see if it would work for you. For us, however, it is best to start with **PSP**, as far as this can be achieved, and then look at what else may be needed to resolve the problem. This may or may not be the 'four principles'; really it is whatever works for you.

In this case, there is conflict between the health professionals, which seems to have roots beyond this incident, and there is also the patient to consider. It's only possible to use **PSP** if you are willing – if the others involved don't or can't use this method there is nothing you can do about it, other than to use it as best you can personally.

The key people are you, Diane, the anaesthetist and the on-call doctor. Your own feelings are clear – Diane needs more pain relief, simple – but whether there are other feelings (of resentment perhaps?) is up to you to explore, personally. Is the anaesthetist irritable to the same extent with everyone? Diane has explained her pain levels and wants better medication; that is clear enough. However, why the anaesthetist has refused the stronger relief, contrary to normal practice, is a mystery.

Ideally, to work this through so it doesn't happen again, you would need the anaesthetist to use **PSP**. Why is her situation so different from yours? Is there any reason you are not aware of that would explain her doubting the patient's claim to be in serious pain? What key factors are influencing the anaesthetist? It would be a big ask to have the doctor genuinely and openly explore her influences and drives, but if this is a recurring set of circumstances it would surely be worth a try. Failing that, it would possibly help to have a team meeting, ideally chaired by a neutral person, with the express intention of working through **PSP** for everyone: ask everyone, how do you see the situation? Why do you see it like this? Why do you see it differently? What do you bring to it that is different from what others bring? Is it possible to agree a plan for the future that everyone is happy with, or at least can live with?

This strategy could, if necessary, fit with the 'four principles' since it could be positively interpreted with reference to each.

Without knowing more, and trying for a better way forward, I would certainly not report the anaesthetist to her line manager.

SUGGESTION FOR SCENARIO 6.4: APPLY PSP TO THIS SCENARIO PLUS THE FOUR PRINCIPLES

—— SCENARIO 6.5: BREAKING THE LAW? ——

CATEGORIES: CONFIDENTIALITY, LAW, PROFESSIONAL ROLE, PERSONAL ROLE

Darren, aged 20, has been admitted to your unit following a road traffic accident (**RTA**). Darren's car was hit from behind by another car, which was travelling at high speed, at a busy road junction.

Darren is not seriously injured – but he has suffered a suspected neck whiplash injury, mild concussion, bruised ribs and some head lacerations.

Following a period of observation, Darren is expected to be discharged within 12–24 hours.

During the admission process, you discover that Darren has a small bag of cannabis in his possession. You ask him about this and he becomes tearful. Darren begs you not to disclose this to anyone, as he is sure he will get into trouble with the police.

What would you do in this situation? Do you agree with the proposal below?

EXAMPLE PROPOSAL FOR FOCUS: It is proposed that you report this finding to your unit manager.

VANESSA'S REFLECTIONS ON THIS SCENARIO

This is a tricky scenario but, personally, I would probably agree with the proposal if I were in this situation (though only out of necessity). However, I would not want to get anyone into trouble unless it were absolutely necessary. I would attempt to ensure that the suspected substance was locked away in the controlled drugs cupboard asap, which would involve informing the nurse in charge of the unit. Whether the substance goes into the cupboard under his real name, a pseudonym, or anonymously, remains another judgement to be made in this particular situation, but I would not want to take this any further by reporting the matter to the police, for the following reasons:

(Continued)

1. Darren is distressed and needs to focus at this stage on recovering (both physically and psychologically) from a recent **RTA** in which he was injured. I would not want to add to this distress at this point in time as this could be counterproductive to his recovery process.
2. The suspected cannabis in Darren's possession is only a small amount. It is currently a crime to possess cannabis in the UK but the authorities will usually turn a blind eye if this is for personal use as long as there is no evidence of intent to supply others.
3. It is common knowledge that there is no legal duty to report a crime in the UK, although morally others (the police especially) see that there is an argument for doing so under a civil obligation to others. This is what it says on the UK police website:

   > Whilst there is no legal requirement to report a crime, there is a moral duty on everyone of us to report to the police any crime or anything we suspect may be a crime. (www.askthe.police.uk/content/Q514.htm)

4. Because Darren has the cannabis on him, it's easy to assume that this was implicated in the **RTA**; however, the evidence suggests that he was shunted from behind and therefore is unlikely to be at fault. However, it does remain possible that the drug was involved in some way.
5. We have no evidence that the cannabis belongs to him or that he is using it from the information supplied.

Nevertheless, despite all of the above, you do have a legal duty to protect others in the unit from foreseeable harms. You also have a professional duty to maintain a trusting relationship and patient confidentiality.

I would reassure Darren that I have no intention of this being reported to the police, but because the small amount of cannabis is a controlled drug it absolutely has to be removed from the unit, in the interests of others, either by a trusted person, or it has to be locked away in the controlled drugs cupboard and logged as such. It would then be collected and destroyed by the pharmacy department.

This said, you can't just take the drug from him as this would undermine the trust he has in you, and you could also end up (though this is unlikely) liable for theft/trespass actions against both you and vicariously the Trust you are working for.

In the event that Darren refuses to give the cannabis to you, what do you do? Personally, I'm not sure. I would have to reconsider again in light of all the circumstances. He does have choices. I would imagine it is likely he would prefer to hand it over; however, we cannot coerce him to do this, as it is his property at present. Some policies advise threatening to call the police if patients refuse to hand over suspect substances but I find this too forceful and think a better solution could be obtained with discussion, choice and reasoning – coercion should be a last resort when all else fails.

So, I would see my duty not as a law enforcement officer but as a health worker who gives and enables choices, seeking to retain trust, and to reduce potential harms to Darren essentially, but also, importantly, to those around him too.

Note: It may be worth noting that this is a mixed picture in the United States (**133**).

DAVID'S REFLECTIONS ON THIS SCENARIO

Vanessa has summarised the legal position of the health professional in circumstances such as these. Essentially the law, and at least some NHS Trusts' policy, says that you are not obliged to report the patient to the police, but should instead convince him or her to hand over the illegal substance, and then confiscate it. The official advice is that you should report the matter to your line manager, in keeping with the proposal above.

However, nothing is legally binding on you, unless there is a specific stipulation in your employment contract, and even then you can still make an autonomous choice to breach the contract. Which means that **PSP** is of central importance here, since it is basically up to you to decide what to do. Legally, you could do anything from completely ignoring the possession to calling the police immediately. Whatever you do there are risks and potential ramifications for you to consider.

In this case, in my reflection I will focus only on the first **P** in **PSP** and then only on the **person** making the decision, since this is a clear example of the importance and influence of personal judgement. If you smoke cannabis yourself, live in a social environment where its use is the norm or at least acceptable, then you are very much more likely to turn a blind eye than report Darren. On the other hand, if you are strongly opposed to drug use, or you or your friends have had negative experiences with cannabis, then you are more likely to report your finding. Of course this is one factor only – we are all so complex – and your negative feelings about the drug will be part of a fluid mix of other influences: are you protective of others? Do you always seek to respect others' wishes? Are you personally risk averse? Are you a health and fitness advocate? What do your close friends think about drugs? Do you enjoy alcohol and other legal highs?

What matters above all else, it seems to me, is that you are aware that your choice, whatever it is, is a matter of personal judgement – that you have brought part of yourself into the circumstances and created a situation. Whatever you decide to do you could decide otherwise. It is in your personal power to do this.

(Continued)

If I were the decision-making **P** in this case, my instincts would immediately kick in, albeit against policy. Details are sparse in the scenario, however it is clear that a substance, said to be cannabis, has been discovered in Darren's possession. I must assume that Darren has told me that it's cannabis since I would be unable to confirm this other than by look and smell, and even then, not being a cannabis smoker myself, I would not be entirely sure.

My personal view about cannabis is that many people report finding it helpful, and in several ways it is less harmful than alcohol. It does not seem to be implicated in the car accident, and Darren has asked me, tearfully, not to tell anyone. I would want to care for him professionally, attending to his injuries and concussion – I would consider this my clinical role, and assisting a quick recovery and safe discharge a central plank of my work for health in this case. As always, as I am treating Darren I would offer information, education and ask him general questions about his life, in case I could promote his autonomy further, in some way. I would neither focus on nor discuss the cannabis unless he asked me, just as I would not discuss finding a quarter bottle of vodka, a big bag of sugar-coated jam doughnuts or a slew of old lottery tickets in his possession.

I am not a police officer, I am a health worker. If Darren were to ask for help with an addiction I would be able to support him in that, but if not, then whether or not the substance is illegal, the cannabis is not relevant to my care. It is not harming anyone else; I have no legal obligation to report the cannabis to anyone, even if it is currently a crime to possess it. He has very clearly asked me not to tell anyone, and is upset both by the accident (he's probably in shock) and by the fact that the cannabis has been found, neither of which he suspected would happen.

I would look to promote his autonomy by helping him recover, by reassuring and calming him, and by giving him space to think about what to do next, or even just to sleep and rest in order to get him back on his feet. I would not tell the unit manager and simply concentrate on a smooth discharge for Darren.

SUGGESTION FOR SCENARIO 6.5: APPLY PSP TO THIS SCENARIO PLUS THE LAW

—— SCENARIO 6.6: BABY SHAMBLES? ——

CATEGORIES: CONSENT, CONFIDENTIALITY, PROFESSIONAL RELATIONSHIPS

Rachel is a 38-year-old married woman. She's been admitted to your unit to undergo a laparoscopic sterilisation.

Rachel has three children, all of whom are under 16. Rachel and her husband – Anthony – have jointly decided that they do not wish to have any more children, especially as Rachel has developed uterine fibroids, which could complicate any future pregnancy. Rachel has tried all forms of contraception, but wishes to be sterilised, as she dislikes the side-effects of medications, and her husband dislikes using condoms as an alternative.

You are the senior practitioner in charge of the unit. As part of pre-surgery assessment you routinely ask Rachel to give you a sample of urine in order to carry out a pregnancy test. This is something that all women in their reproductive years undergo before surgery.

Much to your surprise, the sample comes back positive. You repeat the test, but it still comes up positive. The pre-assessment documentation notes that Rachel suffers from erratic periods, which are sometimes later than expected. Rachel's last menstrual period is documented as six weeks ago.

Rachel's due to go down first on the list that afternoon. You inform the surgeon of your findings. The surgeon says impatiently that the theatre staff are already on the way to fetch Rachel for theatre. He points out that the patient clearly does not want any more children, and he is therefore happy to go ahead.

You promptly inform Rachel of the result of her pregnancy test. Anthony's already gone home to attend to other priorities, so Rachel is on her own. She appears shocked by what you tell her, but very quickly says she doesn't want any more children and is happy to go ahead. You ask her when she will discuss this with her husband. She looks slightly uneasy but quickly shrugs, 'He's in meetings all day and can't be reached. He'll be fine with it. I'll tell him tonight.'

Five minutes later the theatre staff arrive to take Rachel to theatre. You inform them of your findings too, but the staff say they've been ordered to take Rachel to theatre anyway. At that point, they ring the theatre department and moments later the surgeon arrives. He's cross that Rachel is still not on the trolley and accuses you of delaying the theatre list, which will affect everyone. He tells Rachel he's quite willing to take her for her sterilisation – she just needs to get on the trolley.

However, operating on a patient who is pregnant (as Rachel may be) has risks. For example, it is possible that the pregnancy could be ectopic, or there could be issues with the placenta, both of which might increase the risk of bleeding out.

It would also be sensible, and is recommended in some guidelines, to do a blood test to confirm or refute the result of the urine sample. Some would argue that an ultrasound test should also be performed in case there's an enlarged uterus, which might make the surgery more difficult. And according to the Royal College of Paediatrics and Child Health:

> It is generally accepted that elective surgery should be avoided during pregnancy, and that recommendations are required for the anaesthetic and surgical management of emergency situations in pregnant patients. (**134**)

There is also an argument that Rachel has not had sufficient time to process the information, and certainly has not been able to have a discussion with her husband (assuming that he is the potential father).

What would you do in this situation? Should the operation be delayed? Do you agree with the proposal below?

EXAMPLE PROPOSAL FOR FOCUS: It is proposed that you block the surgeon and the theatre staff from taking Rachel to theatre.

VANESSA'S REFLECTIONS ON THIS SCENARIO

There are some key questions to ask here, in order to clarify the **situation**, at least as it appears to you.

Do you think the surgeon has gone through a comprehensive informed consent process in regard to this extra information? Are the circumstances free from pressure? Does Rachel know what alternative options she has? Time is a real issue here – what else could be done to give her extra time to process the information in her own way?

And what about the husband? While there is no legal right for the husband to know does he have a moral right to be informed at least, in your opinion?

Also, the diagnosis of pregnancy needs to be confirmed by a lab test, and I would also want an ultrasound scan done before I would agree to be a part of this, considering she is to have abdominal surgery. The pregnancy – if confirmed – could be implanted in a fallopian tube, for example. If so, then surgery to the abdomen would be even more risky to Rachel and the foetus.

She has consented formally to sterilisation but has she received sufficient information to give informed consent for a termination?

What if she changes her mind?

If it were me, I could try to stop the theatre team physically, but I might get hurt in the process. However, I believe Rachel should be given more time to think about the **situation** and she might change her mind.

Rachel might be making a snap decision because she is anxious about her husband's reaction. However, he might be surprised and feel happy about it. It's also important to consider whether Rachel wants her husband to know, we can only assume that he is the father, after all.

In conclusion, I feel that Rachel would be making a decision to abort the baby under stressful circumstances and without having time to consider the full implications. Being sterilised and having an abortion are two completely different procedures and should not be lumped together into 'one operation'. Furthermore, she has time to make an informed decision with the involvement of her husband and then still opt for an abortion/sterilisation. Or, she might decide to keep the child and be sterilised afterwards.

I would actually block the surgeon and theatre staff on this occasion, verbally, though this is far easier said than done.

DAVID'S REFLECTIONS ON THIS SCENARIO

In this case I agree with Vanessa. Yes there is an argument that she and her husband have firmly decided not to have any more children, but Rachel is in a stressful position, has been presented with new and surprising information, and needs time and space to process what has happened. She needs, in other words, an appropriate amount of time to think through her new **situation**, and the job of a health worker is to free her from pressure, to help liberate her decision-making potential.

In particular, it is important to note that a sterilisation is different from an abortion – some would see it as fundamentally different. The sterilisation is carried out on the woman alone whereas the abortion is undertaken on both the woman and the foetus. Rachel came to the hospital for a sterilisation and, in my view, she really needs time to appreciate the difference and to explore her options with her partner.

This said, if she refuses to take time to reflect then this choice should be respected, but she does need to understand the differences between the procedures, and the risks involved.

SUGGESTION FOR SCENARIO 6.6: APPLY PSP TO THIS SCENARIO PLUS THE ETHICAL GRID

— SCENARIO 6.7: COGNITIVE COMPETENCE? —

CATEGORIES: COMPETENCE, CAPACITY, SAFETY, RISK

You are a health professional working in a busy clinic.

One of your registered colleagues and friend – Susan – who is senior to you, mentions that she thinks she's 'put her back out again' while lifting some grow bags in her garden, but says it will pass: 'it's just a bit of muscle pain, I've had it lots of times before'.

You ask Susan if she feels able to complete her shift or whether she needs to see a doctor, but she assures you she's fine and doesn't want to leave the team short-staffed, as there's such a large caseload of patients to see today. She explains that her doctor has previously given her Diazepam and Tramadol for muscle spasms associated with this issue, which is localised to the facet joint.

Susan is on the waiting list for a Facet Joint Denervation procedure, due to be carried out in the next couple of weeks. She says her medication's at home and she didn't take it this morning, as she knew she was on shift today and her back 'wasn't too bad' when she got up.

During the shift, you enter the room where the staff lockers are. You witness Susan taking medication from her bag. You ask what she's taking. She says 'just a bit of Diazepam and Tramadol, to get me through the shift'. She looks embarrassed, telling you she thought her pills were at home, but she found some in her bag. She then briskly exits the room and carries on with her shift.

You're concerned that Susan is taking medications that could impair her cognition, and she has a caseload of 10 patients to assess today. You pull your colleague aside at the first opportunity. You say that in your opinion she should go home as the drugs she has taken

(Continued)

are very strong and she may not be able to concentrate properly. Drowsiness can obviously affect safety. Susan laughs and replies that she's fine, and to stop making a fuss. She says she takes these tablets often and is quite used to them – it's not a problem.

You are still concerned that your colleague may be putting herself and others in potential danger. Susan made a medication error last week and while no harm was done on that occasion you're concerned that a mistake could happen again if she is under the influence of Diazepam and Tramadol.

What should you do? Do you agree with the proposal?

EXAMPLE PROPOSAL FOR FOCUS: It is proposed that you raise a formal concern over this issue.

VANESSA'S REFLECTIONS ON THIS SCENARIO

There are a number of issues in this scenario which would make dealing with it challenging:

a) A medication error took place the previous week, which involved your colleague.
b) There is a real danger of assumptions being made with regard to the previous drug error.
c) The person concerned is a work colleague and a valued out-of-work friend. This will make dealing with the issue personally challenging, and you may feel very uncomfortable with reporting it to the manager.
d) There is a prima facie legal and ethical duty to protect both staff and patients from foreseeable harms, though these duties always need to be balanced in context. The key question to decide here is, 'is Susan dangerously impaired or placing herself or others at undue and foreseeable risk?' Let's not forget that she also has a back issue and it may simply not be safe for her to work if she is in acute pain and has sustained an injury.
e) The unit is already short-staffed, so there is a potential staffing problem to consider if Susan can no longer work.

This is how I would respond to the health professional who describes the issue above.

First, I think it is important not to make assumptions on the medication error – it could have been an error that any of us could have made under certain circumstances. We must take into account that the previous error may have been unrelated to Susan's medication and back pain. However, I must also bear in mind the possibility that it was related – at this point there is not enough information to judge.

Second, there will more than likely be an element of intuition involved. If you've not noticed anything to be concerned about in Susan's behaviour – either in or out of work – then you may intuitively feel that it isn't really a big deal if she is used to the drugs and her injury. Many people take prescribed medications at work and it does not necessarily mean they are or will be impaired. But were something to go wrong, and you had not reported your concerns, things might look and feel differently.

Personally, I like the idea of talking to my colleague again first, privately and away from the ward area, in a concerned way. Does she need any support? Is this medication prescribed? For how long has she been taking it? In this way, more information may come to light.

It is also important to be frank, making sure she understands what is at stake, as she has legal, professional and ethical accountabilities to her patients, her colleagues, the profession and to herself.

If I feel that if she were impaired then I would be inclined to let her have the opportunity to go home of her own volition, or speak to the manager herself, as she would then be taking personal responsibility for her own actions and omissions. If she were reluctant to do this, and I could understand why (it's difficult for all of us to admit our limitations especially if it means we would be letting our team down), then this would raise a bigger concern for me.

If I were going to inform the manager then I would inform my colleague of my intention to do this, following a more involved discussion.

Safety would be an issue if Susan leaves the ward – voluntarily or otherwise – since it will then be understaffed, but this would be for the nurse in charge to sort out.

Susan may also be cross with you for picking her up on this issue, and may spite you for this in the future. However, I think she needs to know what the facts are and what the consequences may be for everyone potentially involved, explained in a compassionate and supportive way, so she can make her own informed choice.

I would also encourage Susan to see the Occupational Health nurse or her GP as soon as possible, to get signed off sick, if she is judged to be not fit for work. If she still declined to leave the ward or seek clinical help then I would initiate the sick leave myself, while documenting the steps taken to allow her to make her own decision, which she declined.

Susan may need additional support, which would be the ideal outcome from this situation: she may lack insight; she may be in denial about how this medication and her dependence on it is affecting her (although she may still have tolerance and may not be obviously impaired at all).

Overall, for me, the key issue here is about encouraging self-awareness and awareness that there are multiple, contrasting ways of looking at these circumstances.

DAVID'S REFLECTIONS ON THIS SCENARIO

In this scenario the key concepts are **situation** and **plan**. The person recounting the circumstances sees one **situation** – potentially a dangerous one – while Susan, it appears, is taking her prescribed medication, and sees the **situation** as normal for her.

I am assuming that the doctor who prescribed the drugs did not sign her off sick and that Susan is taking the recommended dose. If this is the case then – if I were the **person** observing Susan I would have to ask myself – am I overreacting? Has Susan exhibited other signs of distress or distraction? There was a medication error last week but we do not know what caused it.

If I were the less senior nurse in this scenario, and I was concerned for patient safety, then I would make a **plan**, which would be, as soon as possible, to try to establish a) if Susan is taking the recommended dosage, b) if there is any connection between the medication and last week's error and c) to ask if she needs more support or feels unsafe. If the answer to a) is yes and b) and c) no, then I would do nothing else, other than to reflect on why I feel so anxious about the situation I see – in other words, I would focus on my own self-awareness.

SUGGESTION FOR SCENARIO 6.7: APPLY PSP TO THIS SCENARIO PLUS RISK ANALYSIS

——— SCENARIO 6.8: COVERT CARE? ———

CATEGORIES: CONSENT, CONFIDENTIALITY, PROFESSIONAL RELATIONSHIPS

You are a health professional working on an acute mental health inpatient unit. One of your patients is a 52-year-old woman called Lisa.

Lisa is single and has been unemployed for three years after being made redundant from her job as a hotel receptionist. Over the past two years she has made several attempts on her life while suffering from severe depression. One of these resulted in a lengthy spell of hospitalisation.

Lisa is currently a voluntary patient on your unit. Over the last few days Lisa has been refusing her medication, which she feels does nothing to help her. She says she feels absolutely helpless in her situation.

You observe that the senior nurse on duty – who is also your mentor – has been concealing medication in Lisa's food.

What should you do? Do you agree with the proposal below?

EXAMPLE PROPOSAL FOR FOCUS: It is proposed that Lisa is told about the covert medication and the senior nurse is reported to her line manager.

VANESSA'S REFLECTIONS ON THIS SCENARIO

In this scenario Lisa feels no sense of hope, sees no benefit in her medication, and is therefore refusing to take it. Although to feel despondent is a common symptom in depression, it may be the case that what she's feeling about her medication and treatment is completely reasonable. If, for example, she's been taking the medication for a long period and has not felt any improvement then her refusal is understandable.

The nurse administering the medication probably feels concern for Lisa and most probably also thinks that staff are acting in Lisa's best interests, to help her feel better. However, the nurse's actions are depleting Lisa's choices, self-determination and liberty, and this could make Lisa feel worse, were she to find out.

There's an assumption that Lisa does not have the capacity to understand the implications of not taking the medication. But if so then it is best practice for this decision to be evidenced (in line with the Mental Capacity Act (**MCA**)) (**135**) and discussed and agreed collectively with the Multidisciplinary team (**MDT**) responsible for her care.

There are essential questions that need to be asked in this case study, since the scenario does not make it clear what procedures have been followed prior to giving the covert medication:

- Is there doubt over Lisa's capacity to decide over this specific issue?
- If there are doubts, has Lisa had her capacity enhanced with information, choices, and ways of assisting her to understand? Has this been attempted?
- Has Lisa been offered alternatives and the time and space to explore these?
- Have Lisa's concerns and preferences been listened to and discussed with her?
- Has she received a Mental Capacity Assessment?
- Has this covert medication intervention been discussed, agreed and documented appropriately with the MDT?
- Are the medications being given still being signed for on the drugs chart and clearly stated as being covertly given?

There is a very good reason for policy for covert medication as it must be strictly controlled and monitored to prevent staff from potentially abusing what could be a very dangerous practice. If there were no control this could too easily lay open the path for other staff to secretly give patients sedatives to calm them down for an easier shift, for example, when they are short of resources and manpower. If it's not documented and several staff are using the practice, how do we know whether a patient is being accidentally overdosed?

Above all, each of us has the right to accept and refuse medication, if we have capacity, no matter how ill advised others think our decision is. We also have the

(Continued)

right to know what we are being given. This may have a massive impact on Lisa's care in the future if she were to find out. She may start refusing food for fear it has been tampered with and this will only perpetuate any feelings of paranoia and mistrust arising from her severe depressive state. There will also be a subsequent loss of trust and rapport. Self-determination should not be taken away from another so easily and represents a deprivation of liberty to me in this case. This is why the MCA exists, to protect patients from this kind of practice. Put simply, if we have the ability to decide then we have the right to refuse any intervention, no matter how benevolent the intent, even if it is in our best interests (as others see them).

Assuming that Lisa has had no say in this practice and does indeed have capacity to this decision, I would inform the nurse's line manager and ensure that this covert practice is explained to Lisa sensitively, to try and minimise any harm. This would be in line with a professional duty of candour, an ethical duty of veracity and a legal duty to gain informed consent. Incident forms should also be completed, and everything should be clearly documented.

DAVID'S REFLECTIONS ON THIS SCENARIO

In this case I would apply my theory of health, which describes and explains my purpose as a health worker. According to this philosophy, a health worker should focus on what I have called 'the foundations for achievement' for any person or group she's caring for. In practice, this means that the health worker should create a platform, which can be visualised as a stage on which to perform or move, to support the patient – to make her as strong and equipped as possible.

The key elements of this platform are 'meeting basic needs', 'providing information', 'offering education', 'building a sense of belonging' and, additionally, meeting clinical needs. Constructing and maintaining the main platform is the health worker's primary role, the point of which is very clearly to 'create autonomy' or to empower the patient. The aim of making a strong platform is to place the patient in a position where she can make her own choices, as freely as possible.

Concealing medication radically subverts the proper intent of working for health, and I most certainly would neither do this nor condone it, for this reason. There are several other considerations of course, but for me this is an abdication of a duty to work for health. I would calmly explain this to the senior nurse – and give her some reading materials – and tell her to stop the medication immediately. If she does not I would most definitely report her.

SUGGESTION FOR SCENARIO 6.8: APPLY PSP TO THIS SCENARIO PLUS ANY OF THE CLASSIC APPROACHES YOU THINK FIT

SCENARIO 6.9: PERSONAL OR PROFESSIONAL?

CATEGORIES: PROFESSIONAL RELATIONSHIPS, PROFESSIONAL ROLE

You are a first-year health professional student. You've been working on an inpatient unit as your first clinical placement.

You're caring for an elderly widowed female patient, called Caroline.

You feel you've really connected with Caroline, who's the only patient allocated to you for the day. In fact, you feel you have come to know Caroline pretty well already.

Caroline had to undergo an X-ray procedure. She confided to you that she was very nervous about it, so you personally escorted her to the X-ray department, chatting all the way to minimise her fears.

You go to say goodbye to Caroline at the end of your shift. She thanks you profusely for caring for her, and tells you that she could not have had the procedure without your care and compassion. She fills in her 'friends and family test' evaluation, praising you openly on the form.

Caroline then hands you a slip of paper with her email address on, and asks for your personal email in return. She says she really wants to hear what happens during your career, and she'd love to see how you're doing generally with your life.

You are flattered by Caroline's compliments and wonder if it would do any harm if you gave her your email address.

What should you do? Do you agree with the proposal below?

EXAMPLE PROPOSAL FOR FOCUS: It is proposed that you give your personal email address to Caroline.

VANESSA'S REFLECTIONS ON THIS SCENARIO

I would probably give Caroline my email, but not while there is a professional relationship, even if it were the end of my shift. I would explain to her that I would be glad to hear from and converse with her via email and that she

(Continued)

could write to me once our professional relationship had ended and she was at home.

I would not want to cause her any offence either, because patients do like to express their gratitude. And I do think it's a shame when sometimes staff feel they can't keep in touch with patients they closely connected with. But I do understand why others would have concerns about this.

In establishing some personal boundaries (no matter how flattered I was) I would also explain that this would be as friends and that I wouldn't be able or willing to give her health advice, as that could have repercussions for both of us. I would explain, however, that I would be happy to discuss more general issues and tell her how my life is going. To me that wouldn't be a problem.

DAVID'S REFLECTIONS ON THIS SCENARIO

My 'fast thinking' is, immediately, that I would have no problem with this, so long as I wanted Caroline to keep in touch with me. If I didn't, I would politely decline, and might make an excuse about 'official policy' in order not to hurt her feelings.

I have no doubt that various institutions have various policies about this, and if the one I was working for had prohibited this then I would have to take this into account, as I thought more slowly. But, even so, after reflection, I take the view that this is Caroline's choice as a person and my choice as a person – she is not defined by her status as a patient and I am not defined by my job.

A more extensive 'slow think' might cause me to reflect further about potential negative outcomes, or on Caroline's motivations, or some other nuance, but if she and I want to be friends then that is fine by me. As in all friendships matters will evolve, and further judgements, down the track, will be necessary.

SUGGESTION FOR SCENARIO 6.9: APPLY PSP TO THIS SCENARIO PLUS YOUR INTUITION

——— SCENARIO 6.10: DO YOUR DUTY? ———

CATEGORIES: PROFESSIONAL ROLE, LAW, POLICY, DUTY

Jimmy, a 25-year-old man who suffers with Bipolar Disorder, was admitted to the mental health unit voluntarily a week ago. He has reported increasing depression and suicidal thoughts. He says he has become very socially withdrawn, and has been deliberately isolating himself from his family and friends.

As one of Jimmy's health carers, you feel it's imperative that you're able to build a therapeutic alliance with him. Trust and rapport will help Jimmy communicate openly with you, and also enable you to establish, with the team, his suicide risk.

Jimmy smokes heavily, and although there's a no-smoking policy in operation within the Trust, due to an effort to increase the physical health of service-users, Jimmy frequently visits 'the square' outside, which sits within the unit, to have a cigarette.

On this particular morning Jimmy is restless. When you ask what the problem is, he says he has no cigarettes. You're a smoker, and in your quest to get closer to Jimmy, and to get to know him better, you offer him one of yours and ask if he would like to share a cigarette with you in the square.

Jimmy agrees, and so you're able to establish some trust with him. You share some personal details and he begins to disclose his worries to you.

Later that day you are sternly reprimanded by your manager, in front of Jimmy. The manager says she is extremely disappointed in you for 'getting too close to your patients professionally, and for breaching hospital smoking policy'.

You go home and feel tearful. You feel that you have been totally misunderstood, and that your intentions were clearly benevolent. You feel you were acting in the best interests of your patient, yet you have landed in trouble for your efforts. You don't want to return to work the following day, as you know the manager will be on duty again. You feel you want to speak with her in a way to convey your thoughts and feelings but you do not know how to go about this. You feel unsupported.

There are many conflicts here. How should you deal emotionally with the conflicts between your personal, legal, professional and employment duties that this scenario reveals?

POSSIBLE DUTIES

1. **You have a professional and contractual duty to put your patients' best interests first.**
2. **You have a personal duty to listen to and uphold your own personal values.**
3. **You have a duty to adhere to Trust policy under contractual law.**
4. **You have a professional duty to treat your patients as individuals and promote person-centred care, and to value what they value.**
5. **You have a duty to adhere to the law of the land.**
6. **You have a professional duty not to over-step your professional boundaries.**
7. **You have a professional duty to actively promote health and well-being.**
8. **You have a legal and professional duty to provide safe care and to minimise risk to service users.**

Do you agree with proposal below?

EXAMPLE PROPOSAL FOR FOCUS: It is proposed that DUTY 2 is the most important duty in this situation.

VANESSA'S REFLECTIONS ON THIS SCENARIO

My instinct is to give Jimmy a cigarette and try to get him to open up to me a little, after establishing some trust. Whether I would actually smoke with Jimmy I don't know, that would depend on other factors; I might just decide to sit with him. Some staff would be less understanding than others and this might make me reticent to actually sit and smoke with Jimmy, especially if I were working with individuals who might berate me for it. But on the plus side, to be able to summon up the courage to do this with Jimmy, would be a connection made and some common ground established.

I realise that what I am saying may be shocking to some; however, this would be a natural response to a person in need, in my view. I have looked at both sides of the spectrum regarding this scenario, and attempted careful 'slow thinking' to explain my reasoning. My choice represents an autonomous, free-thinking decision at the right pole of the spectrum, though it is a complete deviation from hospital policy, current anti-smoking health promotion strategies, and the current EU legislation it derives from. This I am aware of.

It's very important to listen to, question and if we still value them, uphold our personal values, where justified. We need to listen to our intuitive feelings and preferences where possible, especially if we feel our integrity is being questioned, tested or breached. If I get an anxious feeling, a hunch or a strong feeling to do one thing or another, I tend to ask myself why I feel that way, and then make a further judgement based on that.

Enabling Jimmy to have a smoke outside, although not ideal for his physical health and safety, gives him choice and may help build up a more therapeutic relationship which could improve his long-term mental health. There's a slight risk to others around us in this public area, but those people are there by choice to smoke. However, this doesn't mean that we don't have a duty to them. I would want to move away from others and find somewhere quiet in the square to sit with Jimmy. Others might also think it odd if they see one of their health professionals smoking with a patient, so that would go through my mind also. Maybe I would wait a while until the square was empty.

This strategy, for getting a connection with a patient in this group is not uncommon. It's well recognised as an effective way of establishing common ground, rapport and trust with others, aiding communication in persons who may feel isolated in themselves. Some may be shocked to know that it was not unusual (historically) for patients who were in hospital for weeks upon end to be wheeled out by their nurses for some fresh air, a chat, and (ironically) a cigarette. I have even done this in the past with young patients who are on traction for serious trauma injuries. I think anything that assists communication, and assists with the assessment process, is beneficial, on balance, especially in a potential suicide case. However, it also has to be acknowledged that mental health patients have a poor level of physical health, which has been attributed to smoking. There are drives in place currently to try and improve the physical health of these groups of people, a demonstration of this is a ban on smoking in and around mental health units. I personally do not agree with this move, I think it's unsustainable, no matter how well intentioned, since it misunderstands the complexity of addiction behaviour and its underlying causes.

I also need to bear in mind that I am a smoker, a bias if you like. I'm not sure if I would feel any different if I wasn't, it's impossible to say. I think I would empathise with Jimmy anyway, since the last thing I would want, if I were in his position, is somebody taking away my only support, even in the form of a noxious cigarette. Smoker or not, I think I would feel that my liberty was being further eroded. I think I might even feel trapped in an over-paternalistic pseudo-prison as a result.

Of course, there are plenty of people who would disagree with sharing a cigarette with Jimmy, both smokers and non-smokers alike. When polled on the Values Exchange, the issue always splits 50/50. The most common reasons cited against sharing a cigarette are 'a blurring of boundaries', 'he may expect preferential treatment in the future', 'it's against Trust policy', and 'it's bad for his physical health'.

There are also now new EU laws governing smoking in hospital grounds, which, as we see, strongly influence local Trust policy. It is also true that in the current ethos it would not be seen as professional to give patients cigarettes and share them.

For me, however, this is about context and specific situations. A blanket approach does not respect individuality or meet individual needs, nor is it person-centred care. By making Jimmy my priority I would be willing to take the possible disciplinary consequences because the benefits outweigh them.

I would document my justifications for deviating from Trust policy. It is true that breaking Trust rules and sharing one of your own cigarettes may be stepping over the sometimes difficult to identify personal/professional boundary, but sometimes we need to give a little to gain a client's trust. It must be very hard for a client who is a heavy smoker to cope with their mental health problems while 'detoxing' from nicotine – something I'm not sure I'd have the strength to do when feeling as low and vulnerable as Jimmy does at present.

In this scenario, for me, **DUTY 4** most closely reflects my own personal philosophy of how I would see work for health in Jimmy's situation.

This scenario and the one above, about Caroline and the email, both concern professional boundaries. I understand that some may see my observations as contradictory: isn't giving an email address (which I would not do while at work) less significant than sharing a cigarette with a patient at work? However, I see these scenarios quite differently. In Jimmy's case, the boundary issue is secondary to me. Of much more importance is the fact that Jimmy has a real clinical need for someone to establish a level of trust with him, as soon as possible, to allow him to open up so that he can be properly assessed.

DAVID'S REFLECTIONS ON THIS SCENARIO

To set this as a question of conflicting duties is a really interesting approach, and highlights just how much of everyday decision-making is not only beyond the rules, but beyond simple logic. Each of these duties is effectively a rule. Not only do you ultimately have to select at least one of them to make your choice but you also have to use your judgement to decide what each means and then, somehow, weigh them in order of importance. The duties cannot speak for themselves.

Should I adhere to my personal values or should I deny them? To answer this I need to know what my personal values are. And I also need to consider other factors. This decision – like every other healthcare decision – is not merely an analytic, logical process of deciding which value trumps all the others. It's a personal, partly unpredictable voyage.

I know I am strongly in favour of creating and respecting autonomy in the people I'm responsible for at work – which points me in the direction of having a cigarette with Jimmy, for the reasons the 'you' in the scenario give. But not only do I have more than one value, like everyone else I am a complex person, shaped by all the forces in **Figure 4.2** and more. I would be affected by several of these in this case – not least 'peer pressure' and 'social history'. Were I to sit in the square and have a cigarette with Jimmy against policy, in the knowledge that most or all of my colleagues would disagree with me (which let's face it is likely) then I would feel awkward and self-conscious at best: I would be going against the group, which human beings find very hard to do. I am aware that the largest part of my personality is to do exactly this, certainly it was when I was a young man, but I would not want to alienate my colleagues or risk personal repercussions either, even though I'm sure there's no harm to anyone else caused by a couple of cigarettes in the open air. Another part of my personality, which has grown stronger over the years, is to go along with things I find mildly wrong rather than cause a big fuss. Which part of me should be dominant and how do I decide?

What I need to work out overtly, as a slow-thinking calculation, is what is in Jimmy's best interests (conformity? suicide prevention? happiness? health – whatever that means?), what I personally value most (supporting patients in their wishes? keeping my job? doing what really matters to me?), which law to follow (adults have a legal right to smoke, hospitals have a legal right to try to stop them), being 'person-centred' (do I do what Jimmy wants or do I try to protect him in another sense?) and much more. And beyond this calculation I need to **feel**, in a personal way, what is right. What, if anything, would feel emotionally and physically most right to me?

I think, though I am not certain, that after considering all these factors steadily, I would do what the 'you' the health professional – in this scenario would do, even in the knowledge that I would be potentially endangering my career by so doing.

I would be aware that other staff would disagree with me and prefer me to adhere to policy, and would have their reasons for this. Other staff might even feel shocked and possibly undermined by my choice. But I would have good reasons for wanting to use 'talking therapy' with Jimmy, and helping him relax and gain trust by sharing a cigarette with him. If by doing this I could reduce his suicide risk, and help him feel more positive, then I would feel justified (of course I do not know if my actions would actually have this effect, but I would want to try, since there is a chance that they would).

While sharing a cigarette I would create autonomy by respecting Jimmy, listening to him, talking to him, spending time with him, informing him, educating him and as far as possible empowering him to cope better with life. I see that as my rationale as a health worker. I have written in favour of this consistently and at length and – while I am always reflecting and always open to revising my views – I would act out my theories in practice, aware of the reasons and feelings behind my choice, and the potential negative consequences. Going against my values and rejecting **DUTY 2**, would, to me, have worse negative consequences because I would feel inauthentic. (**136, 137**)

SUGGESTION FOR SCENARIO 6.10: APPLY PSP TO THIS SCENARIO PLUS VALUES-BASED DECISION-MAKING

— SCENARIO 6.11: CONCEALED BULLYING? —

CATEGORIES: COMMUNICATION, CONFLICT RESOLUTION, MENTAL HEALTH

You are a health professional working on a busy Mental Health Unit.

While checking your off-duty rota you notice that an early shift you had previously requested has been changed to a late shift, without your knowledge. You specifically requested an early on this particular day so you could attend an appointment with your General Practitioner.

The senior nurse in charge of the off-duty rota has failed to communicate this change to you. This is something you've noticed happening more frequently lately, since you returned to work four weeks ago, following a long period of stress-related sick leave. The senior nurse in question is perceived to be stern and authoritarian by yourself and some of the other team members. You've found her to be unapproachable and inflexible whenever you've attempted to discuss off-duty concerns in the past.

The ward has been very busy of late. There are also high levels of stress-related sick leave amongst other staff. As a consequence, some staff have been asked to change

(Continued)

their shifts and cancel annual leave at short notice. Although this has created some degree of disharmony and frustration amongst the team, most have been flexible and accommodating, including yourself, with any changes, in the interests of placing the patients and the unit first.

At the moment you feel upset and angry. You're increasingly feeling that you are being personally targeted by this senior nurse, as evidenced by the lack of communication with you, which she clearly affords to the other members of the team. You're becoming more and more convinced that you are being covertly bullied, due to your recent long period of stress sickness, which left the ward under-resourced.

You are not sure how to resolve this issue or how to cope with your feelings.

What would you do to resolve and effectively manage this perceived conflict?

Having identified your emotions and feelings, why do you think these emotions are occurring? You may wish to consider past experiences and your personal values. What is important to you?

What possible reasons can you think of which may account for the senior nurse failing to communicate with you lately?

What do you think would be the best time and place to deal with this conflict?

How do you think you could help resolve this issue in a collaborative way and avoid this conflict escalating further, and what would you say?

What do you consider to be the potential consequences of facing this conflict as opposed to not facing it, and using avoidance tactics instead?

EXAMPLE PROPOSAL FOR FOCUS: It is proposed that you make a formal complaint.

VANESSA'S REFLECTIONS ON THIS SCENARIO

This situation is one which comes up quite frequently. I have experienced or witnessed many versions of this in the past, and so can relate somewhat.

I have experienced having my shifts changed last minute without being asked. I have had plans and had to cancel them, as there has been no one else to cover. It is very frustrating and has made me feel undervalued, on occasions. I feel it is important to be flexible but at the same time such changes should be communicated to prevent upsetting members of staff.

The nurse in this scenario may feel victimised as she recently just came back from long-term sick leave, and sense that she is being blamed for leaving the ward short-staffed. She may also feel frustration in the heat of the moment because she's requested time off to go to see her GP, but her request has been ignored.

The nurse in charge may take the view that she is merely trying to do her best to cover the ward's needs. But if it were me, I would not feel comfortable or feel valued enough. This is not the first time and many questions would cross my mind. Is she doing this because I have been off sick or is she genuinely doing her job in the best way she can?

It would be important for me to try to have a calm and private conversation before I can decide what to do next, but the prospect of confrontation would cause me anxiety, since she appears unapproachable. Her rationale may include any one or any combination of the following. She:

- values your work
- is trying to punish you
- has poor communication skills
- forgot to communicate with you
- is genuinely trying her best to cover the ward
- feels envious of you for some reason
- has a desire to control
- is being strongly pressured from above
- is suffering from the effects of burnout and stress
- has a lack of self-awareness
- values your flexibility

I think it's important to try to understand everyone's motivations as soon as possible but it's also important to wait until raw emotions have settled and there has been time to reflect. It's all too easy to fly off the handle, and the danger is that you might then act upon assumptions that may not turn out to be true.

Conversely, it's also important to be true to yourself and if you truly believe you are being treated unfairly or your integrity is being breached then it's important to raise this, speak up and try to resolve it.

I would like to be understanding towards the senior nurse's **situation**. After all, she is struggling to cover shifts due to many team members taking stress-related absence from work. I would, perhaps, offer to alter my shift patterns to help. I would also consider changing my GP appointment if this were a real emergency and no one else could possibly cover the shift.

In this case it is really important to work as a team – to understand what the nurse in charge needs and for her also to understand the conditions you work in – to try to see each other's situations, in other words.

If this perceived conflict were to continue, despite a conversation, then I would document evidence, seek witnesses, professional advice from HR or a union, and

(Continued)

consider raising a formal grievance (if all else failed). I have found that if you do address these conflicts directly with the person involved, one to one, the negative behaviour will usually reduce; not always, but mostly. Often, the 'bully' is not aware of the effect they are having on others, especially in times of stress, and can be genuinely surprised to discover the impact of their behaviour on others.

DAVID'S REFLECTIONS ON THIS SCENARIO

This is an interesting scenario because it focuses directly on **situations**, which of course are the **S** in **PSP**. The key to resolving this scenario – if resolution is possible – is somehow coming to view different **situations** at once, in particular the senior nurse's **situation** and your own. There are obviously different perceptions going on, caused by complex relationships at several levels, and so while there are certain objective facts there are also different **realities** in play. We all know this just from life experience; however, my experience is that we tend to forget it or underestimate it and end up believing – often unshiftably – that our **situation** is the objective reality and everyone else has got it wrong, or is more or less deluded.

Of course, if there are facts that are not known by one or more of the people involved, these should be introduced. For example, does the senior nurse know the cause of the stress 'you' have suffered and which caused you to take such a long sick leave? If she does not then there is a chance she will be more sympathetic if you – or someone else – calmly informs her. Do you know what else is happening in the senior nurse's life to perhaps cause her to be antagonistic to you? Again, it would be worth trying to find out.

If there are no further facts – though life is so complex there always are, it's just not always so easy to discover them – then the focus should be on trying to achieve some sort of empathy (though as we discuss elsewhere, in **Chapter Four**, there are significant difficulties with this concept).

What I think should happen is a meeting between 'you' and the senior nurse, facilitated by a person you both trust. This would not need to be a long meeting but it would allow you both, perhaps, to change your **situations**. If you felt able, it would be a good idea for you to say openly that you have looked at your emotions and past experiences and wonder if you are colouring the present circumstances in an unhelpful way, and also to say that you do feel uncomfortable and 'could we all openly look at why this should be?': a sort of mutual counselling session.

There is no guarantee that this would help and it might even make things worse, but this is what I would recommend.

It is extraordinarily difficult to place ourselves in another person's shoes, and even harder to be honest with ourselves about why we are who and what we are, and why we are behaving as we are now.

SUGGESTION FOR SCENARIO 6.11: APPLY PSP TO THIS SCENARIO PLUS WHATEVER ADDITIONAL MEANS OF REFLECTION YOU SEE FIT

SCENARIO 6.12: CURRENT ACCOUNTABILITY?

CATEGORIES: PROFESSIONAL ROLE

Doris is an 80-year-old woman who's been admitted to your unit due to an exacerbation of Chronic Obstructive Airway Disease.

Doris is expected to be on the unit for at least 7 days.

You are a health worker on the unit. While attending to Doris and her fundamental care needs, Doris explains that she has direct debits due to go out of her current bank account in the next 24 hours. She has a cheque in her bag that she was about to deposit at the bank, the day she was admitted to the unit.

During this conversation, Doris asks if you would be willing to drop her cheque in for her after your shift, so her direct debits are not declined, and to avoid expensive bank charges.

Doris does not have any family or close friends who are able to do this for her. It turns out that you both share the same bank, and you were planning on going into town after work anyway.

Do you agree with the proposal below?

EXAMPLE PROPOSAL FOR FOCUS: It is proposed that you pay the cheque into the bank for Doris, after your shift.

VANESSA'S REFLECTIONS ON THIS SCENARIO

To prompt reflection, I first present an anonymised response from a health professional posted on to the Values Exchange in 2017. This judgement contrasts with my own and, although I don't agree with the professional in this instance, I feel it's well worth including as an example of a well-reasoned, balanced and justified reflection, as follows:

(Continued)

As an individual in a caring profession, I would personally want to help and support Doris as much as possible. As this issue is causing Doris a lot of anxiety, and affecting her respiratory rate and effort, I feel that saying no to Doris would increase her anxiety levels further, but this would be unacceptable for me to do as I would have access to Doris's bank account, and if the cheque was not paid in properly, or the money went missing, then I would be responsible and would lose my job.

Even though this proposal makes me feel uncomfortable, I would still want to support Doris as much as possible. I would offer to refer the case to social services, and explain to Doris that even though this may take a while, I would explain that it is an urgent matter and if the bills are not paid in time, I would ask social services to possibly contact the companies to make them aware of Doris's hospital admission.

The consequences of carrying out this proposal would be if the money went missing, or any money went missing from Doris's bank account, I would be held responsible for this, and may risk being prosecuted. If I did carry out this task for Doris, I would ensure that I obtained receipts to prove that I had paid the money in to show that no money had been taken out of the account by myself.

Even though I would be off shift, I still have a duty of care to protect my patients, and also to protect myself. I would feel that I would be placed in a vulnerable situation by transferring money into a patient's bank account, and there may be consequences if anything goes wrong.

The most compassionate person-centred thing to do, is to explain to Doris that even though I would have happily transferred the cheque into her bank account, I would be in serious trouble if anything happened, such as money going missing. I would explain to Doris that I will refer her case to social services as urgent, as they are able to deal with financial matters, and support her with her anxiety levels, and explain that she does not need to worry as her bills will get paid. I will advise her that I will ensure social services will deal with this matter as quickly and efficiently as possible, and the main priority is getting her better and helping her to recover.

In this reflection piece I particularly like the way that the health professional has tried to balance Doris's needs with her own. She clearly wants to help Doris but is honestly fearful that she will get into trouble if she does. She's acknowledging that she simply would not be prepared to put her own job on the line to do as Doris asks. Although I think this is a shame, I get the impression that, in an ideal world, she would very much like to have the freedom to help.

The professional applies some useful reasoning, even if I do not agree with her final judgement. The professional looks for solutions such as involving Social Services and suggests getting them to ring the companies involved on Doris' behalf.

However, despite the positives here, there are some points in her reasoning with which I don't agree:

- The professional says that if she does as Doris asks then this would be a breach of confidentiality. This simply is not the case. Doris has given explicit consent to share her accounting information with you, and therefore confidentiality between you and she does not apply, though sharing her details with others, without permission, probably would.
- I would not personally feel this matter is worthy of referring to Social Services. Although it may be put through as an urgent referral, they may not see it that way. From experience, most Social Services referrals take days to put into action, because of limited resources. I would want this issue addressed asap, which is why I would be inclined to pay the cheque in for her, to minimise harm to her psychologically, physically and financially. I think the risks are minimal. It's simply a deposit, which can be made with a sealed envelope and even deposited through the cash machines outside the bank. A receipt of deposit can also be obtained.
- There is no professional or contractual duty of care to patients when off shift, only within the course of employment. Unless you were in uniform (which could be interpreted as being in the course of employment) then the duty you have to her is a personal one only. There is a civil duty, under the tort of negligence, to avoid acts and omissions that may impact on someone who is close enough for your acts or omissions to affect them. There is also a civil and criminal duty not to steal or be fraudulent when dealing with other people's property.

Other options available to help Doris could include, if she is well enough, Doris calling the banks and companies involved herself (very difficult if she is short of breath) or for you to do this for her, with her explicit consent of course. Again, she would be sharing private information with you. There might be someone, a friend maybe who could help or maybe it would be an option to get the accounts department involved.

I see this as totally in the remit of a nurse's role, although others may disagree. I feel sad when issues like this come up because it just seems like common sense to carry out this simple task, yet the risk is often seen as far too high, when it's actually minimal compared to the risk to Doris of not carrying out her wishes. However, I do acknowledge that risk-averse approaches exist to protect employees and are sometimes necessary, but I worry for the person-centred care lost in the process. In my experience of caring for people with these types of worries, no amount of reassurance will help Doris until the issue is actually dealt with, as she wishes, in a swift and timely manner.

DAVID'S REFLECTIONS ON THIS SCENARIO

My fast thinking tells me that there is no problem with my doing this. It is simply a kindly act. I am aware that there are perceived issues with befriending patients – see **Chapter Three Myth Three** for example – however, I do not think it's a problem. I see emotional reaction to others as a human inevitability. Of course, just as you would not want to show negative emotions or hostility to a patient you dislike, you should avoid being over-friendly to those you do like. You should also behave consistently, and you should establish boundaries, for example by explaining to Doris that this is a one-off because of the circumstances. Otherwise I really see no reason why you should not do this simple favour for another human being.

SUGGESTION FOR SCENARIO 6.12: APPLY PSP TO THIS SCENARIO PLUS THE ETHICAL GRID

—— SCENARIO 6.13: A BITTER PILL? ——

CATEGORIES: CONSENT, LAW, PROFESSIONAL ROLE

Julie, a 20-year-old hairdressing student was diagnosed with paranoid schizophrenia a few months ago. She has now been admitted to the Acute Mental Health ward, detained for treatment under Section 3 of the Mental Health Act 1983 (amended 2007) following an episode of acute psychosis.

According to both staff observations and reports from Julie's concerned parents, Julie is exhibiting more frequent and increasingly violent outbursts, hyper-sexuality and delusional behaviour. This escalation has coincided with Julie's decision to discontinue her antipsychotic medication.

One night, after the lights are dimmed on the ward, one of the nursing staff discovers Julie in the toilets with a male patient, having sexual intercourse.

Julie is not on the contraceptive pill and it is established that the male patient did not use any protection during this event.

The following day the nurse-in-charge obtains a prescription for the morning-after pill for Julie. There are concerns from medical staff that if Julie becomes pregnant then this will affect her treatment options and chance of having a successful remission from her psychosis.

As a support worker, you're present when medication is being checked for administration to Julie. The charge nurse, who is your mentor, checks the morning-after pill and pops the tablet into the medicine with Julie's other medication.

The charge nurse checks Julie's identity band, then gives Julie the pills without explanation, which she takes without question. It quickly becomes clear, following a discussion with the charge nurse, that Julie was unaware that she was given a morning-after pill and that this was done covertly in her 'best interests' without informed consent.

What would you do in this scenario? Do you agree with the proposal below?

EXAMPLE PROPOSAL FOR FOCUS: It is proposed that you inform Julie that she has swallowed the morning-after pill.

VANESSA'S REFLECTIONS ON THIS SCENARIO

There are three obvious **persons** in this scenario, however the outcome of this issue has wider potential implications for others on the unit under the care of this Charge Nurse.

Even though Julie has previously been sectioned under the Mental Health Act (**138**) there is no information stating that she currently lacks capacity to make this particular decision, and therefore capacity must be assumed in law in the first instance (**135**).

Arguably, healthcare workers have both a moral and now, more recently, a legal duty of candour (**139**) to be honest with service users, to foster trust and openness between professionals and service users. However, this must also be balanced with preventing further harm to Julie, so any disclosure must be made sensitively and compassionately.

In this incident, information should have been given to Julie about the potential consequences and risks of her and others' actions, and she should be offered education about sexual health, enabling her to make informed choices. Having said that, she may already be well aware of this and still chose to engage in sexual activity on the unit. It's also important to ensure that there was no coercion involved in this sexual act while Julie remains under section on the unit, and therefore vulnerable. The Trust and the professionals owe a duty of care to Julie. Julie also needs to be aware of the side-effects of taking the morning-after pill, which may impact upon her.

It is for these reasons that I strongly question the Charge Nurse's actions.

Although the nurse administering the covert medication may think she is acting in Julie's best interest, to ensure that Julie recovers from her acute episode of illness, a clear assumption is being made here. The nurse is assuming that Julie does not have the capacity to choose what she would like to do over an issue that she is not under section treatment for. Julie's freedom and choice has been taken away from her under the guise of paternalism and protection. It is Julie's right to refuse medication for contraceptive purposes and she deserves the same standard

(Continued)

of care under the Medicines Act (**140**) and under informed consent legislation as any other patient in these circumstances.

I agree that, although hard to break to her, Julie should be gently informed, ideally by the administering nurse responsible. I also would want to discuss this matter with Julie and explore her knowledge of sexual health. She will also need psychological support for the breach of trust demonstrated to her by the administering nurse. I think that, again although difficult, the Charge Nurse should be reported to her line manager, having had the opportunity to do this independently.

This should be treated as a serious incident. A plan of action can be made to ensure that this nurse is both educated and supported and learns from this, through reflection and discussion, and that some form of remedial action is sought for the patient involved.

DAVID'S REFLECTIONS ON THIS SCENARIO

This scenario is similar to, though not the same as **Scenario 6.8**. I don't think **PSP** is particularly useful in this scenario, at least not for me. As in **Scenario 6.8** I would see my purpose as 'work for health' and 'creating autonomy', and one of the central foundations of this theory is 'providing information'. It is clear to me that Julie needs to know what has happened.

I do not think the nurse should have covertly medicated Julie – the medication is not related to her condition. I think it amounts to an assault. I would tell the charge nurse what I think and give her some reading about the law. I would also want her to consider how her actions are part of a care plan for Julie, and I would ask the nurse what she sees as her purpose as a health worker, and where she would draw the line in administering other medication without patient knowledge or consent.

SUGGESTION FOR SCENARIO 6.13: APPLY PSP TO THIS SCENARIO PLUS THE ETHICAL GRID

SCENARIO 6.14: A CASE OF MISTAKEN IDENTITY

CATEGORIES: SAFETY, RECORD KEEPING, LAW

You are a newly qualified nurse, working on a paediatric unit. You're receiving handover from an experienced nurse, Ruth, who's just completed a 12-hour shift, her third in a row, due to staff shortages. Ruth complains to you through handover that she's been feeling unwell during the latter end of her shift – she thinks she's developing a possible upper respiratory infection. She also says 'these long days are killing me' and that she 'can't wait to go back to her 8-hour shift pattern after her days off'.

During handover she reports on a child – Mark Smith – who's had a catheter inserted, following an episode of acute retention of urine, after abdominal surgery the same day. Ruth gives a brief handover, as she is keen to leave the unit, and says the rest of his information can be found in his notes, where she's made a comprehensive entry of assessment, interventions and evaluations.

You're assigned to care for Mark during your shift and immediately consult his notes in order to decide how best to proceed with his care. However, you soon realise that there appears to be no entry made by Ruth. You're confused and suddenly realise that there are two patients on the ward with similar names: Mark Smith and Marcus Smith. You decide to check Marcus Smith's notes and you see that indeed a comprehensive entry has been made by Ruth – but for the wrong patient, by mistake.

You're unsure what to do next. What do you think? Do you agree with the proposal below?

EXAMPLE PROPOSAL FOR FOCUS: It is proposed that you report this mistake to Ruth's line manager.

VANESSA'S REFLECTIONS ON THIS SCENARIO

I wouldn't report this myself but I would encourage and support the nurse to discuss the incident with the line manager, to enable open dialogue, to raise concerns and to find some kind of change to the shift patterns this nurse is currently working. I would also try to find ways collectively (as a team) of avoiding this mistake happening again. Even if no harm came to the patients involved, this could have been dangerous and even fatal.

In my opinion, this is both an individual issue and a matter that can be partly attributed to organisational pressures and the low resources available – which makes longer shifts seem more attractive. Long shifts have been associated with low staff morale and a higher incident of mistakes occurring (**141**).

Some nurses are able to tolerate long shift patterns and prefer them; however, others are quite the opposite, and prefer 8-hour shifts in order to feel they can practise to their full potential, and with the due diligence that those under their care expect from them.

This nurse is clearly tired and becoming ill. She suffered a moment of inattention which led to a genuine mistake, partly due to lack of ability to concentrate and partly due to the conditions and context she has been working in.

(Continued)

I would invite Julie to rectify the entry at the earliest opportunity in line with Record Keeping Guidelines. RCN guidelines state:

In the rare case of needing to alter a record, the original entry must remain visible (draw a single line through the record) and the new entry must be signed, timed and dated. (142)

I would also recommend that she complete an incident form. If patient care has been affected in any way then I would encourage her to also file an additional incident form. Health professionals are also encouraged, under a duty of candour (139), to be open and honest, explain what has happened to those involved, and also apologise to patients, relatives and carers – even if no harm occurred. It is recommended that professionals still do this if there was only a risk of harm. There's a risk that the organisation you work for may want to discourage you from doing this (in order to protect themselves from complaints or even claims of liability if harm occurred). However, Trusts can be prosecuted by the Care Quality Commission (CQC) if they do not adhere to the new statutory standards, and nurses can have their registration questioned if they fail to explain mistakes, even if no harm occurred.

Moving forward, I would ensure that if there were two service users of a similar name being cared for at the same time, this should be made well known and acknowledged by all clinical staff. I would also encourage practitioners to speak up if they feel they cannot operate at a safe level on 12-hour shifts, and feel they are becoming emotionally and physically burnt out in the process.

DAVID'S REFLECTIONS ON THIS SCENARIO

I would not report this to the line manager. It is a perfectly understandable mistake and could have happened to anyone in the trying circumstances staff are experiencing.

Even though I have less experience than Julie I would be at pains to support her in raising this at the next team meeting, at the top of the agenda, and also, once Julie has agreed, advise the formal measures Vanessa describes. This is obviously a matter that not only could have happened to anyone but which affects everyone – both staff and patients. There is a paramount need for openness, candour, honesty and disclosure – and it's for the team as a whole to work together to ensure that nothing similar occurs in the future.

SUGGESTION FOR SCENARIO 6.14: APPLY PSP TO THIS SCENARIO PLUS THE NMC CODE

SCENARIO 6.15: NOVICE VS EXPERT (ADULT VERSION)

CATEGORIES: CARE OF THE ELDERLY, DEMENTIA

You're a third-year student nurse working on a very busy Care of the Elderly Unit. It's your first day. The Senior Nurse is showing you around. After a quick orientation she tells you you'll be shadowing a Senior Health Care Worker. 'Remember' she says, 'I expect the ward to be straight by lunchtime!'

While you're both walking down the nightingale-style ward, you're stopped by an 82-year-old woman, who's sitting beside her bed. She grabs hold of your trousers and pulls you closer, asking, 'What's the time?' 'What's for lunch?'

She keeps hold of your trousers firmly. But before you can reply, the Senior Nurse states loudly and impatiently, 'Mrs Smith's demented. She always asks the same questions. She won't remember anything you say. Come on dear, you've a lot of work to do. She'll have you there all day.'

What would you do?

EXAMPLE PROPOSAL FOR FOCUS: It is proposed that you do as the Senior Nurse instructs you.

VANESSA'S REFLECTIONS ON THIS SCENARIO

My gut reaction is a feeling of shock and injustice towards this patient. I would feel uncomfortable excusing myself from her when she so obviously wants to converse, but I would also worry about the senior nurse's reaction if I stayed: she may be cross and angry with me, possibly in front of the patient, which would make the patient feel uneasy too.

Overall, this situation would make me feel very awkward but I would hope my personal values would uphold and I would have the courage to be true to myself as an advocate. I would hope to be able to say that I would come back and speak to this

(Continued)

lady soon, but I would also address her immediate questions and possibly have a conversation with the senior nurse in private. This would be very difficult in reality.

The strength in this proposal is that if followed it would, I suspect, keep the senior nurse happy and I would naturally want to fit in with and be accepted by the team on my first day, and make a good impression. However, the weakness is that I would be ignoring this lady's request for information and reassurance. To stay and converse would be to meet her needs, but I would fear the wrath of the senior nurse if I did. I would perceive her to have more knowledge and experience than I, not to mention power and control, so I would be putting myself at risk of reprisals if I ignored her order.

The senior nurse's obvious motivation to 'get straight before lunch' and 'come on we have a lot of work to do' makes me think she's more focused on tasks than engagement. From my actual experience I have seen this many times: the ward looks tidy and ordered, with every patient sat out and washed at the same time. But this is not necessarily a well-run ward.

I have been on wards where the beds may not be perfectly made, and there's paperwork everywhere, but when you look more deeply the patients are happy, content and chatting to each other and the staff in a meaningful way. Not everyone is washed at the same time, not everyone has their breakfast at the same time, not everyone goes to bed at the same time, and individuality is respected.

I think that sometimes nurses may distance themselves from patients in this way so that they can tick off the boxes and say they have got their jobs done in time, and maybe this is also a way of not suffering the pain which comes from empathising with a patient. Targets and tick boxes only serve as a means to an end, yet the process is just as important as the goal. It is not so much for me about **what** we are doing but **why** and **how**.

Furthermore, to label the patient as 'demented' serves only to depersonalise her and define her needs as irrelevant. It's likely to result in nurses disengaging with her, since they realise the senior nurse perceives it as a waste of valuable time, which can be better spent on other tasks.

The reality, from experience, is that most persons with dementia have periods of complete lucidity, and recognising these instances and times actually shows that we're taking notice of them in a 'person-centred' way.

The nurse/health carer–patient relationship is complex and involves power. The patient is usually vulnerable and, therefore, in a weaker position than the health carer/nurse, whom the patients tend to see as holding special power and knowledge. Most patients are unwilling to challenge the clinicians since they risk being labelled as 'difficult' or 'confused', or worse. Nurses and health carers must always be mindful to try to find the person behind the label – as well as any underlying concerns which have not been identified – by engaging with and getting to know the patient's story.

Having the courage to speak up is also important in this situation. It should not be assumed that because someone is senior to you they necessarily know what's in the best interests of the patients. Of course, having the ability to stand up and do what you value has to be balanced with fitting in with a team. This requires integrity, communication skills, advocacy and the willingness to display attitudes and behaviours that may challenge the ward culture. In this way, compassion stands a chance of flourishing and patients can be facilitated to be autonomous decision-makers, as far as possible.

DAVID'S REFLECTIONS ON THIS SCENARIO

If I were the junior nurse I would be very torn in this situation. I would instinctively want to stop and talk to the patient, but just as instinctively I would fear negative consequences for myself. I'm not a nurse in reality, but I do have a lot of experience in ethical reflection. So I think and hope I would stop and tell the elderly lady 'I will come back with answers as soon as I can', and then I would follow the Senior Nurse.

I would return as soon as possible. This would be respectful and also enable me to make a personal assessment of the patient and her needs.

SUGGESTION FOR SCENARIO 6.15: APPLY PSP TO THIS SCENARIO PLUS THE NMC CODE AND SIMPLE RISK ANALYSIS

CHAPTER SIX EXERCISE

Pick a reflection from either David or Vanessa with which you disagree, and use whatever method of reasoning you prefer to explain why.

CHAPTER 7

PRACTICE SCENARIOS: PATIENT AND FAMILY ISSUES

SCENARIO 7.1: MARIE — TO LET GO OR NOT?

CATEGORIES: RISK, RIGHTS, DUTY, POLICY

It's a very cold icy morning. There's been a surge of people coming into the A&E department of the hospital where you work with various degrees of injury because they have slipped on ice.

Marie, a 40-year-old woman, has been admitted onto the day case surgical ward. Marie suffers with anxiety and depression and is awaiting elective surgery to explore and repair a suspected torn medial meniscus (knee fibrocartilage tissue). Marie was dropped off by her husband because she does not drive.

Due to unforeseen circumstances within the theatre department, Marie suffers a long wait prior to surgery. She eventually becomes frustrated at what she perceives to be a lack of progress and communication as to when she will be taken for her operation. Suddenly, after waiting 4 hours, Marie gets up from her chair and limps purposefully down the corridor, stating angrily that she is 'sick of waiting' and she wants to 'go outside for a cigarette'.

The hospital Trust in which you work operates a no smoking policy within its buildings and grounds. The hospital has very large grounds and to leave the grounds entirely would require at least a 15-minute, painful walk for Marie, who is unsteady on her feet.

What would you do in this scenario? Do you agree with the proposal below?

EXAMPLE PROPOSAL FOR FOCUS: It is proposed that Marie be prevented from leaving the ward to have a cigarette, prior to surgery.

VANESSA'S REFLECTIONS ON THIS SCENARIO

EU law has stated that smoking is now prohibited in hospital buildings and grounds. This is reflected in individual hospital policy. It's difficult, however, to see how this can be enforced, or even how a practitioner can advocate for a patient's preference to smoke, without considering prevention. There's a definite risk to the practitioner of disciplinary action should she respect patient choice and escort her outside for a cigarette, not to mention the potential wrath of the surgeon.

In this case, a patient has become very frustrated by insufficient communication. She should have been kept informed in a more proficient manner, she should have been put earlier on the list, and she should have been offered nicotine patches or other alternatives. It's quite unreasonable to expect someone who smokes to give up smoking for a day in hospital, no matter how physically damaging it is to them: this lady is seeking comfort in a coping mechanism to deal with a situation she feels upset about.

We should have talked calmly to her about the risks, options and alternatives prior to surgery, and that she may miss her slot if she's found to be outside smoking. Ultimately, however, whether we like it or not, her current mood and attitude is a reaction to our failings, as she sees them, and the fact is that we have no legal, professional or ethical right to stop her from leaving the ward. She's not in a secure unit or in prison, and to coerce her or physically block the door could result in a claim of trespass, assault and deprivation of liberty.

A clear part of a nurse's role is to promote health, and this is endorsed by the profession. But in doing so we also have to pay attention to the psychological health needs of patients. Indeed, some benefit might come from allowing her to have a cigarette. She would be calmer, and less likely to increase her anxiety levels and, therefore, her blood pressure. It is obviously not what I would see as a standard health intervention, but there are some perceived benefits here potentially for Marie.

Marie, if she decides to go for a cigarette, is at risk of falling if she has to walk to a smoking area. Giving her a wheelchair or assisting her could reduce this risk. There's also a slight risk to the general public of 'passive smoking' if she chooses to smoke within the grounds. And there's a danger to the organisation if something were to happen to her while off the ward, if unaccompanied. In the end it is her choice – we can only inform, and then it is up to her to make her choice as a competent adult.

In my opinion, a nurse's role is to inform, educate and empower. It's not to be an enforcement officer or to pass our value judgements and opinions on others. Marie values others things differently from 'official policy', and these values should be respected where possible, if we are to be meaningfully person-centred. Blanket bans of this and that, while well intentioned, do not reflect the fact that we're all individuals, and in this sense they can actually produce more harm by disempowering persons.

DAVID'S REFLECTIONS ON THIS SCENARIO

My experience of using this scenario in teaching sessions revealed both the value and the limitations of the **PSP approach**.

In workshops with four groups of third-year pharmacy students, each independently decided that, if at all possible and within the law, Marie should not be permitted to leave the ward – even to the point (for two of the groups) that she should not be told the truth that she has every legal right to do so and cannot legally be physically prevented from leaving.

At first I found this rather amusing, expecting that when the students had thought about it more clearly, they would realise that there are ethical and logical difficulties that would cause them to change their minds. But the more I challenged them the more I could see the situation through their eyes, and the more I was caused to question my own 'obvious' judgement. But this is surely the value of **PSP**.

(Continued)

I don't smoke (Vanessa does) but I seem naturally to gravitate towards the view that if a person wants to smoke then that is her choice, just as it is her choice to drink alcohol or eat fatty food – so my perspective in this regard might be called 'libertarian' or at least in favour of supporting personal choices even if I disagree with them (of course it's much easier to support those I do agree with!). So my view – or my situation – sees a frustrated person, increasingly needing a cigarette being pointlessly prevented from having one due to an excessive focus on one small risk above all others (i.e. smoking is bad for health, therefore we can't allow it in a hospital – nothing else matters).

The students' situation was framed very differently. They felt that she should not walk 30 minutes to the edge of the hospital and back: a) because this would be painful; b) because it might further damage her knee; c) there is a risk of falling; and d) she might miss her turn on the theatre list. She needs the op so we should support her in waiting patiently for her turn, they decided. This is best for her health – it's a bigger harm to miss the op or to have it delayed than it is to miss a cigarette for a few hours, they saw. Our job, they said, is to talk and support her, to enable her to cope without cigarettes for as long as it takes – creating longer term autonomy.

They did not consider – or more accurately did not even see – the alternatives, like helping her have a cigarette in the grounds, driving her to a safe place for a smoke with an instruction to the hospital staff to call the mobile if her turn comes up, challenging the policy as illogical and unlawful. This view was simply not seen, just as I had not seen their view: their **situation** and mine were mutually invisible. Put another way, my specific values and theirs, in this instance, were not just different, they were incompatible.

I find this realisation fascinating, instructive and disconcerting. I am now much less sure that I would be right to help her find a place to smoke, but this still remains my inclination, for now.

SUGGESTION FOR SCENARIO 7.1: APPLY PSP TO THIS SCENARIO PLUS VALUES-BASED PRACTICE

SCENARIO 7.2: DNR TATTOO – HELP OR HINDRANCE?

CATEGORIES: EMERGENCY, COMMUNITY

You are a Community Nurse, on a routine visit to Aarav, a 33-year-old patient, who has had surgery for testicular cancer. His cancer has spread to the retroperitoneal lymph nodes in the back of his abdomen, for which he is receiving chemotherapy. Despite this spread the cancer is highly treatable, with a 5-year survival rate of 96% (**143**).

Aarav has been extremely upset about the removal of his cancerous testicle. He says even with reconstructive surgery his 'manhood' has been permanently damaged. Aarav has recently ended his long-term relationship with his girlfriend. He told her he knows she wants children but that is now very unlikely since he decided, without telling her, not to store any sperm.

You are monitoring Aarav's physical and mental health, and have been particularly worried that he appears increasingly depressed.

On this visit you knock to gain entry to Aarav's flat, and as you do so the door swings open. Aarav is unconscious on the floor in the hallway. You quickly notice that he has an empty packet of prescription opioids in his hand, and his shirt is open at the front. On his chest is a colourful tattoo, which says, in large letters:

DNR

And under this the instruction:

I do not want to be resuscitated under any circumstances.

The tattoo is dated one week before the date of his surgery, but is apparently neither signed nor witnessed.

For those individuals who strongly desire not to be resuscitated, the tattoo idea is appealing. By its nature, a tattoo implies a preference against resuscitation so strong that the person has etched the image onto their body. The tattoo is inseparable from the body. Unlike Do Not Resuscitate (**DNR**) paperwork or medic-alert bracelets, it cannot be misplaced, easily removed, or lost. Emergency responders are unlikely to miss seeing a **DNR** tattoo on the chest prior to attempting resuscitation.

Clinicians are legally obliged to respect the preferences of patients to forgo life-sustaining treatment. However, in the absence of written and witnessed paperwork such as an advanced directive, is a tattoo enough? What if the person has changed their mind recently or in the past and has not had the tattoo removed? What if the tattoo is a joke? Or it refers to a rock band? What if there are no family or friends around during an emergency to clarify wishes on behalf of the patient if they are unconscious? And even if family and friends are around how do you know that they are accurately conveying the patient's wishes? Do they have other motives? And in any case, their advice to you on behalf of the patient has no legal standing.

Given all this, what should you do? Do you agree with the proposal below?

EXAMPLE PROPOSAL FOR FOCUS: It is proposed that you ignore the DNR tattoo and immediately call an ambulance.

VANESSA'S REFLECTIONS ON THIS SCENARIO

I have found this issue very difficult to decide. It has taken some deliberation, yet a practitioner would have only a few valuable moments to decide, at best.

This appears to be an emergency.

- Aarav has cancer, has received surgery and the cancer has spread.
- Aarav is probably suffering from depression from the effects of a cancer diagnosis, his infertility and major loss of body image affecting his manhood.
- Aarav has a very clear DNR tattoo.
- The tattoo is neither signed nor witnessed but was carried out recently, prior to surgery.
- There is no obvious paperwork to support DNR decision or any witness present.
- Aarav chose not to store his sperm and may be regretting this now.

My first and natural inclination, due to my personal philosophy, would be to uphold and respect this man's wishes. I am a great believer that people should have personal choice and self-determination over what happens to their bodies. I would feel very uncomfortable jumping on Aarav's chest to resuscitate him for example, given his overt DNR tattoo. If he were to be successfully resuscitated (by the attending health professional or emergency services) he would probably feel very distressed if he genuinely wanted to die, and may descend into an even deeper depression.

Having said this, after careful but swift thought and deliberation, I changed my mind about this scenario.

Despite being a person who values a person's autonomy and choice, I would ring the emergency services and probably attempt life-saving interventions for the following reasons:

- Aarav may have been aware that the nurse was due to visit imminently and, therefore, this may be a genuine cry for help.
- Aarav's cancer is highly treatable.
- Aarav did have a long-term girlfriend. He may now be making a false assumption that she won't be able to love him due to his perceived loss of manhood and infertility issue, knowing that she wanted to have children in the future.
- There are surrogate/adoption/foster/sperm donation opportunities for people who have become infertile from cancer treatments, who want to have children with current or future life partners.
- Aarav appears depressed. Has he received any form of therapy/medication for this? Has he had the opportunity to speak to others in a support group who have been through similar, successful treatment for testicular cancer?

Aarav may see his situation as hopeless, despite the high treatment success rate associated with this type of cancer – he may fear that it's just a matter of time before it comes back again, even if given the all clear. This is common for patients who have gone through cancer treatment. They tend to fear that they haven't been told the truth.

- This event was not foreseen or expected.
- I am aware that a person who has taken an overdose of opiates or narcotics can be successfully resuscitated under some circumstances with the administration of Naloxone (**144**).

If Aarav were to be rescued he would have the opportunity to explore the points set out above and may well seek assistance and retain some hope for the future, being able to live a full and active life once again with a loving partner by his side. Therefore, although I wouldn't be completely comfortable, in this instance I would ignore the tattoo.

Finally, if Aarav is intent on committing suicide I don't see that there is anything anyone can realistically do to stop this from happening if they are determined, and sometimes this is completely unforeseeable and unavoidable – persons sometimes keep their personal feelings very private, even away from their loved ones. I have seen this happen from personal experience. A colleague lost a parent to suicide, and no one saw this coming. The parent had recently been given the all clear from cancer, and while the family were celebrating this good news, committed suicide only a week later. My colleague (who was a nurse) didn't foresee this. It was a complete shock to everyone, since the parent was widely perceived as brave, outgoing and positive. This highlights the isolation and the private personal struggles those who have gone through cancer and its treatment sometimes experience. It seems that even when the prognosis is good, we can never be sure what someone is dealing with in their own reality.

DAVID'S REFLECTIONS ON THIS SCENARIO

It is difficult to form an instant opinion on this situation, but in real life one would have to. For some reason, in this case, 'fast thinking' doesn't happen for me.

I think, to be honest, that my natural inclination is to try to save Aarav, but I am immediately conflicted too: he seems to be wanting to die and has made this as clear as he possibly can, though there is no mention of a note.

I know – or at least I think – that legally, since this is an emergency, it would be lawful to try to resuscitate him, since the tattoo is not witnessed and may not be genuine. But I am personally torn. The philosophy of health I believe in tells me I

(Continued)

should try to 'create autonomy' – that is, I should try to help Aarav and give him the opportunity, if he can be saved, to think again. And I would do everything I can to support him in this, but at the same time, I have my own feelings about the value of life, and do sometimes see it as futile, so I would also feel justified in walking away.

I would find it hard to apply **PSP** to this issue, too.

Thinking as quick as I can, I would try to resuscitate him, reluctantly.

SUGGESTION FOR SCENARIO 7.2: APPLY PSP TO THIS SCENARIO PLUS YOUR INTUITION

──────── SCENARIO 7.3: NO ENTRY? ────────

CATEGORIES: SAFEGUARDING, EVIDENCE, LAW

Joanne, a 23-year-old female, was admitted to the Medical Assessment Unit three days ago, due to vomiting and diarrhoea of unknown origin. She was dehydrated on admission and received intravenous fluid replacement. Tests have found no cause for Joanne's symptoms, but she has improved a little over the last 24 hours and is due to be discharged in the next day or two, once the results of a stool sample have been received.

Although Joanne appears to have decision-making capacity, she has some developmental delay and learning difficulties, and appears rather immature for her age.

Joanne's long-term boyfriend Adam has been attending the ward frequently and staying for long periods, sometimes out of routine visiting hours. You've noticed that when Adam's on the ward he tends to speak for Joanne and tries to make her decisions for her. You've also witnessed him looking at her phone while she's asleep and using remarks that could be interpreted as intimidating.

Adam has been overheard making comments like, 'Wait till I get you home, you'll have your work cut out then', ' Are you sure you're not just trying to get out of the house work by being in here?' and 'Hurry up and get better – washing's piling up and no-one's there to cook my tea.'

He's also commented, directly to staff, that Joanne's lazy and 'probably poisoned herself ... to get out of her responsibilities'. Although this seems to be said in jest, you're concerned that Adam displays little compassion and deliberately undermines Joanne's confidence. This is apparent from Joanne's posture and demeanour when he's around. Joanne also seems more withdrawn and anxious than usual whenever Adam is due to visit.

Joanne doesn't receive any other visits, from either friends or family, and seems heavily dependent on Adam, who's described Joanne's family as 'misfits' and was once overheard saying that Joanne would be 'better off without them'. Joanne says she fell out with her family and some of her friends while living with Adam, because they didn't like him. She says they're probably jealous of her close relationship with him.

Joanne gave up her job as a receptionist at her local GP surgery three months ago, in order to be a housewife, which Adam apparently encouraged. Joanne says she misses work but wants to be 'a perfect housewife' for Adam who, she says, 'works very hard' and 'deserves to be cared for'.

While helping Joanne in the bathroom you notice heavy bruising to her left upper leg, and her upper arms. When she sees you looking, Joanne quickly covers up. Naturally you ask her how she got her bruises. She responds, 'oh it's nothing, I fell on the stairs last week. I bruise easily'.

You feel concerned both about the bruising and about Adam's attitude towards Joanne. You've spoken to your team leader and you've raised the idea that it might be better for Joanne if Adam is prevented from coming on to the ward. Joanne has not asked for this and has said 'he loves me very much, he's only joking in what he says you know'.

You ask her directly if she would prefer him not to be allowed on the ward, at which she becomes agitated and upset, rejecting the idea with 'no, he must be able to visit, he will be upset if he can't'.

What do you think? Is the proposal below a good idea?

EXAMPLE PROPOSAL FOR FOCUS: It is proposed that it is in Joanne's best interests for Adam to be prevented from entering the ward area, while the team further investigate the situation.

VANESSA'S REFLECTIONS ON THIS SCENARIO

This proposal would make me feel uncomfortable for several reasons. On the face of it, it seems logical to stop Adam from entering the ward in order to protect Joanne. I would naturally feel protective towards Joanne since at first glance it seems she is most likely being exploited or abused, either psychologically or physically or both.

However, when I look closely at this issue I think we have to be very careful that:

a) We do not make assumptions or base our actions or omissions on assumptions which have not been confirmed or validated by Joanne, as a competent adult who has capacity, despite some learning difficulties.

b) In an effort to protect Joanne we do not reduce her autonomy further by disregarding her wishes or making choices and decisions for her which would reinforce her feelings of low self-worth when she is discharged into the community, where she will remain dependent upon Adam.

(Continued)

It's easy to assume that Adam is the cause of Joanne's bruising, yet she denies this, and although denial is common in cases of actual abuse (through possible real fear of ramifications, or as a coping mechanism to normalise the situation) she may also be denying it because she actually did fall on the stairs and bruises easily.

I would want to check Joanne's blood values to see if there is any evidence of blood dyscrasia, which may indicate easy bruising. Is she on aspirin or on any medication that may affect her platelet level?

It may also be the case that Adam is 'bantering' with Joanne, and although this may be unacceptable to others and cause concern, this may be normal and acceptable to Adam and Joanne. I suppose my concern is if he isn't allowed to visit then this may well impact on her well-being. She has not corroborated any evidence – the only evidence is what staff have observed.

Certain aspects of this situation particularly need to be taken into account:

- Joanne cannot stay on the ward for an extended period without clinical need, and most cases of abuse would be investigated only with consent of the victim, out of the hospital setting.
- She has capacity and has not said she doesn't want him to visit.
- She may decide to discharge herself if he isn't allowed to visit.
- He may (assuming he's abusing her) abuse her more when she's eventually released, if he feels she's disclosed information to the team. He may, possibly, already have warned her of the consequences if he's stopped from visiting, or if she discusses him with the team.
- She may well refuse to divulge information if she feels intimidated as a primary witness, which is a common occurrence in these situations.

I think the potential ramifications need to be taken into account and that Joanne should not have her stated wishes overridden. An enabling approach should be initiated by providing information and lines of support that she may wish to take up. I think it's important – if she is in fact being abused – that we do not disempower her by taking her choices away from her, since this will likely reinforce the feeling that she has no control over her life or choices. We need above all else to try to enhance her autonomy.

Supervised visits may be the way forward, with consent. But this has to be in a way which doesn't put her in further possible jeopardy when she's eventually discharged.

DAVID'S REFLECTIONS ON THIS SCENARIO

I do not agree with the proposal, mostly because I do not think it's the role of health professionals to act in pseudo-policing roles. This may sound rather harsh and uncaring, but if I were the nurse I would not directly intervene between Adam and Joanne because:

- She has not asked me to
- Evidence of abuse is not definite
- I am not competent to make this intervention (barring Adam) safely
- I am aware that there is a high chance that the consequences for Joanne and others, including myself, could be bad if I intervene between them
- I might further disempower Joanne
- I would consider this intervention beyond my role as a nurse/health worker

Vanessa has explained most of these points above. I would like to focus on the last point – preventing Adam from visiting and otherwise intervening between them would be beyond my role as a health worker. The essence of a health worker's role is to enable – or create autonomy in – the people for whom she is caring. It is an empowering role that aims to give as much control to the people being cared for as possible, so they can make their own decisions. It's not a health worker's role to try to manage broader life circumstances involving other people for whom they are not directly caring for.

I am aware that not everyone would agree with my definition of the role of a health worker. And in recent years there has been a movement towards 'safeguarding' patients beyond simply treating their medical conditions (see for example **145, 146, 147, 148**).

However, there are subtle, but important, differences in these approaches, which may help explain my own judgement. In my view, the 'Making Every Contact Count' strategy, initiated by the NHS, oversteps the line between 'working for health' and coercion. It:

… encourages conversations between staff and clients/patients based on:

- behaviour change methodologies (everything from brief advice to more advanced behaviour change techniques)
- empowering healthier lifestyle choices
- exploring the wider social determinants that influence all of our health …

And:

[Giving] …

Level 1: brief advice and signposting, for example to smoking cessation services, reducing pupil absence from school

Level 2: behaviour change intervention, for example brief intervention, increasing physical activity to target groups

Level 3: behaviour change intervention programme, for example weight management programmes, exercise by prescription (**149**)

(Continued)

An apparently similar, but less coercive, approach says:

> If nurses think a woman in their care may be experiencing domestic violence, the detail of questioning will depend on how well they know the woman and what indicators they have observed. Nurses should begin with broad questions, such as:
>
> - 'How are things at home?'
> - 'How are you and your partner relating?'
> - 'Is there anything else happening that may be affecting your health?'

Specific questions linked to clinical observations could include:

- 'You seem very anxious and nervous. Is everything all right at home?'
- 'When I see injuries like this, I wonder if someone could have hurt you?'
- 'Is there anything else that we haven't talked about that might be contributing to this condition?'

More direct questions could include:

- 'Are there ever times when you are frightened of your partner?'
- 'Are you concerned about your safety or the safety of your children?'
- 'Does the way your partner treats you ever make you feel unhappy or depressed?'
- 'I think there may be a link between your illness and the way your partner treats you. What do you think?' (**150**)

The Making Every Contact Count approach is only coincidentally 'work for health' – it's possible it may promote autonomy but it's more likely to stigmatise and blame people by picking on their supposedly bad habits. If a person is having life difficulties and you wish to help them, then you should first engage them in open, general conversation about their lives and their goals: what is working well for you in life? What is missing? How do you think you might feel happier? What subjects would you like to learn more about? Focusing only on topics like smoking, school attendance, exercise and weight management is arbitrary – why these topics and not poverty, media propaganda, poor school teaching, the meat and dairy industry, or pot holes in the local roads? The latter are just as likely to cause traditional 'health issues' and impact negatively on the NHS as smoking and eating too much.

If people ask for help that is very different from trying to change their behaviours because you – not they – would prefer them to behave differently.

In Joanne's case, while it is not appropriate to prevent her boyfriend visiting her, unless she requests it, it is definitely appropriate to try to enable her to tell you if she is in trouble, and to try to find out if she would appreciate your help. It's definitely appropriate to establish whether she has unmet basic needs you could help with (freedom from fear, for example), needs information, needs help to understand her situation, and whether she would benefit from recognising the range of choices that may be open to her, which you could explain. Doing these things would be potentially autonomy creating, and up to her to request if she wants, whereas giving her your opinion and advice about her relationship and situation without being asked is not enabling her, it's putting her under pressure and stressing her.

The aim of health work is to empower people by giving them as many options and capacities as you can, while treating them with the utmost consideration and respect. It is not the aim of health work to try to convince people to see the world the way you see it.

I would ask Joanne gentle questions, and perhaps leave relevant reading materials nearby. I'd give her opportunities to talk safely. But if she did not want these then I would respect her choice and leave that area of her life alone. (**69**)

SUGGESTION FOR SCENARIO 7.3: APPLY PSP TO THIS SCENARIO PLUS THE ETHICAL GRID

— SCENARIO 7.4: TO VACCINATE OR NOT? —

CATEGORIES: PAEDIATRICS, CONSENT, AUTONOMY

Last month you qualified as a nurse. You now have your first job, working in a health centre at the local private school. Today your supervisor has told you that you are to administer the 3 in 1 booster (Diphtheria, Tetanus and Polio) and the MenACWY vaccine (Meningitis A, C, W and Y) to all 14-year-olds whose parents have provided explicit consent for these injections, in written form, to the school.

Your supervisor is extremely keen on immunisation and tells you that you must vaccinate every child, without exception. She says the science is conclusive – vaccination is safe and in everyone's best interests. She says that sometimes these adolescents get upset and anxious about vaccinations, but if that happens you should just reassure them that all is well and go ahead and inject them.

The same supervisor disciplined another junior nurse recently for refusing to carry out her delegated instructions, and although this nurse is now looking for another job, she is currently finding it hard to work with the supervisor who, everyone agrees, has an authoritarian management style.

You begin your vaccinations for the day. All is going fine until you ask Andrew to roll up his sleeve for the needle. He gets very upset and says that he really doesn't want to have the jab, he's read this up online and doesn't agree with vaccination, despite what his parents say. You ask him to sit down while you check his paperwork, which confirms that his parents have

(Continued)

indeed consented to the jab. You call your supervisor who says you absolutely must go ahead since the paperwork is signed. She becomes annoyed and tells you again to just reassure him and do the injection, as this is what the parents want and they will be upset with the school if this vaccination does not proceed.

You go back to Andrew and tell him he must be immunised. Andrew starts to cry and sob and is physically resisting any contact with you by lashing out and pushing you away with his arms and hands.

He shouts that he is scared and he wants to go now.

What would you do? Do you agree with the proposal?

EXAMPLE PROPOSAL FOR FOCUS: It is proposed that you go ahead and vaccinate Andrew.

(149)

VANESSA'S REFLECTIONS ON THIS SCENARIO

This is a complex issue. There are many people involved in this scenario. The nurse, Andrew, his parents, the school as an organisation, and the nurse supervisor in charge of the vaccination programme.

Let's start with looking at Andrew's parents and the school in question.

THE PARENTS

As Andrew's parents, they have signed a consent form. They have legal responsibility for decisions made about Andrew concerning his health, as he is under 16 years of age. They clearly want him to receive the immunisation.

We can only assume that the information they have been provided with is not biased, and that they have therefore given truly informed consent. Many organisations have targets to reach to achieve herd immunity, and although these organisations may have the pupils' best interests at heart – in that if some don't receive the vaccination then other pupils may be at risk – it is also important to know that many (including schools and the NHS) also receive financial rewards if they reach these targets. Therefore, we must always be mindful of how information has been presented and try to avoid any pressure, misrepresentation of the facts, and to acknowledge inevitable bias. What was sent out to the parents? Was it factual and balanced, or heavily biased in the programme's favour?

My question at this point would be – have they (the school or parents) discussed this information with Andrew prior to signing the consent form? Has he been pressured in any way or not had his voice heard because he is still a minor? Any omission to discuss this issue with Andrew may be behind his distress at this point. Reflecting on my own teenage son, who is a similar age at the moment, I know how much he likes to be involved in decisions made about him and how upset he feels if he thinks he hasn't been consulted.

THE SUPERVISOR

The supervisor is very pro-vaccination and public health. However, there's a danger that the **person** may be lost in the process if the programme runs like a conveyor belt or a production line. 'Everyone must be vaccinated' essentially means that she is working to a standard that she may have created based upon her own beliefs, or based upon the organisation's agenda – that is, the only situation she is aware of is the one she sees.

While there is a clear professional duty to public health, legally we do not have a duty to those who are not proximal to us at the time. The school has a vicarious duty to all the students, but the nurse only to those who are currently in her care – or close enough to be affected by her actions or omissions.

It may also be the case that the supervisor is receiving pressure from the organisation from above to ensure that all the parents are kept happy as far as the pupils' jabs are concerned. In a private school, the parents pay the fees and, up to a point, they call the shots in some ways. From my experience of private education, schools such as this try to keep on the side of the parents as much as possible, after all, they pay the staff wages.

ANDREW

It is obvious that Andrew has strong views in this scenario. He's distressed, he doesn't want the vaccination and says he's read stuff on the internet about it. He is physically and verbally resisting the immunisation, and this would not be easy for him, as he probably would not want to upset his parents, the school, the nurse or cause a fuss in front of his peers.

We don't know how credible Andrew's information is. We also don't know if he's had a discussion with either his parents or the nurse about to vaccinate him – or whether he has just been told to 'roll his sleeve up'.

My intuition in this scenario is that Andrew feels unheard and in a situation in which he feels he has no control, despite his advancing years. It may be that 'Gillick consent' could apply here – if it were to be established that Andrew is clearly able to weigh up all the information and make an informed decision for himself (151).

(Continued)

THE NURSE

Imagining being the nurse in this situation, I would value the individual more than the wider public here – of course, others may disagree.

If a person were physically and verbally resisting an intervention I would want to stop and I believe I would, despite the potential ramifications to me. I would see my duty to Andrew, and I would not want to assault him by restraining him physically or verbally – this should always be a last resort. I would want to build some trust first, and demonstrate respect for his autonomy, as an individual who has a say in what happens to his own body, and who may well meet 'Gillick competence'.

I would want to reassure Andrew and have a discussion with him. I would want to ask him open questions and give him the opportunity to ask his own questions before proceeding with any line of action. I have a duty of care to him, right here, right now, in the present – and only secondarily to the public.

Of course, herd immunity is important, to offer good levels of nationwide protection for all – but at present Andrew may well go ahead with the vaccination anyway, after a little time to settle. My primary concern is to get him informed, to understand and to be heard. He may well change his mind at this point. Even if there is written consent from the parents, who have responsibility for Andrew, anyone is free to change their mind at any point prior to a clinical procedure taking place – even if the parents have the final say, I would argue that even as a minor, it is prudent to ensure everyone is heard.

It's obvious to me that Andrew, the health professional involved, and the parents need to discuss this matter further in light of Andrew's reading and research findings and his trepidation, before any vaccination is given. A discussion should take place which includes all parties as a group, focusing on the benefits, the risks and any alternatives available. It may simply be the case that Andrew has read something which is not from a credible source or it may be that his concerns are indeed legitimate and from a sound source of evidence.

I would explain my reasoning to the supervisor, being mindful of the pressure she may feel under also, but if the supervisor decides to 'make my life difficult' I would also document any incidents, with details of time and place and refer them to the relevant line manager along with my concerns. I would also gain advice from a professional union.

DAVID'S REFLECTIONS ON THIS SCENARIO

This is a 'fast thinking' issue for me. Faced with a young person upset and adamant that he does not want an injection I would not force him. Simple as that. It would not matter to me what age he is, so long as he's competent to make informed life choices, which I am assuming he is, then it is not my role to compel him to have a vaccination. It is not work for health, in my view, so I would instinctively try to calm him down and tell him straight away that I will not coerce him. This would be an instant decision for me, caused both by my nature and personality and by my theorising in health philosophy and ethics over many years.

Of course, I am aware that this is a complex matter scientifically, ethically, politically and legally, and I have researched and written about it at length in papers and books. But in this situation – my **situation**, as I perceive it – there is no time for analysis, nor is it necessary. I will not stick a needle in another human being who is so clearly telling me not to.

I would talk to Andrew, gently and carefully, since I would – as a health worker – want to create as much autonomy for him as possible. This would mean that I inform him of the facts about the vaccination, as far as they are clear, and also, to be fair, tell him that not everyone agrees with it. I would also recommend articles to read – pro and con – and tell him that he should work out why he doesn't want the injection. Is his fear justifiable? Why do his parents want him to have this vaccination? Would it be better just to accept it, or does he feel so strongly that it is a matter of principle?

SUGGESTION FOR SCENARIO 7.4: APPLY PSP PLUS TO THIS SCENARIO USING RISK ANALYSIS AND EVIDENCE-BASED PRACTICE

— SCENARIO 7.5: LOST IN TRANSLATION? —

CATEGORIES: FAMILY ISSUES, CONSENT, AUTONOMY

Sasha is a 38-year-old mother to eight children, living in Birmingham, UK. She has had five caesarean births, the latest only four weeks ago. Sasha does not speak or read any English.

The surgeon who delivered her last baby was able to explain to her and her husband – via an interpreter – that if she were to get pregnant again, the risks to both her and her baby would be extreme. The most likely outcome would be a ruptured uterus, which would be catastrophic for both her and her baby.

Sasha is from a culture where the husband makes all the decisions. He does not believe in contraception and will not even discuss it.

Your final maternity visit with Sasha (supervised by the midwife) is scheduled for a time when her husband will be at work, and you discover that your organisation is unable to make an interpreter available to translate between you.

As a recent immigrant, Sasha has no family support and cannot drive. If you do not discuss her health and birth control options with her now it's unlikely that she will be able

(Continued)

to consult her GP or other health professional without her husband finding out. Sasha's oldest daughter, aged 14, speaks both English and her native language. She is your only way of communicating with Sasha at the moment.

Should you involve the daughter? Do you agree with the proposal below?

EXAMPLE PROPOSAL FOR FOCUS: It is proposed that Sasha's daughter should translate your discussion about contraception for her mother.

VANESSA'S REFLECTIONS ON THIS SCENARIO

This is a very complex issue which raises many issues, difficulties and concerns for me. First, I need to look at the persons involved.

The scenario affects all three (Sasha, the husband, and the daughter) plus the other existing seven children, potentially.

There isn't a lot to go on and ideally I would want more information, so I will have to make some assumptions along the way.

Sasha is at very high risk of uterine rupture and haemorrhage due to her previous caesarean sections if she has any more pregnancies. We don't know if Sasha wants any more children – logistically she simply can't without a high risk of potentially catastrophic consequences for her, her baby in utero, her husband and her remaining children. Becoming pregnant again is not an option here without harm being caused to all. So, there needs to be some kind of preventative measure which both Sasha and her husband agree with, despite the husband's strong cultural beliefs, which we must take into account. I'm sure he would not have agreed with her previous sections if he didn't care and therefore we can only assume that he wants no harm to come to her. If left to nature, the fact is that Sasha and maybe her children would not be alive, so to disagree with other preventative measures would seem incongruent.

It is important to highlight that it is now enshrined in law that health and social care services have a legal duty to provide appropriate communication support to people under the Accessible Information Standard of the Equality Act, including the appropriate use of interpreting services in their many forms.

I do not feel it is appropriate at this point to use the daughter to translate. It is quite possible that something may be 'lost in translation'. There is no absolute guarantee that all the conversation will be effectively translated (there have been many cases of family members only translating what they want the person to hear, and this may even be what has been happening if the husband has been translating for you in the past). In addition, the father may place blame on the child for giving the information to her mother.

A child may not understand the topic being discussed and it seems unfair for this to be the way she learns about her mother's issues. Also, we must not assume that Sasha is happy for her daughter to be present during any conversation, and we must somehow gain her consent before moving forward with any interventions.

It also strikes me that this situation is something that would have been foreseeable – maybe this complex scenario could have been prevented if the antenatal midwifery team or a surgeon had found a way to manage it prior to the last caesarean taking place. For example, a conversation could have happened, with the help of an interpreter, which might have given Sasha the option of receiving a sterilisation at the same time as having the caesarean operation. In Western civilisation, it's usually the mother who has the final say over what happens to her own body, and although this may be in conflict with Sasha's husband's beliefs (we actually don't know how he feels about sterilisation) it is something which is advocated and upheld in UK law, as well as by the majority of Western ethicists. Therefore, every effort must be and should be made to explain things to Sasha and her husband (with consent from both of them) to enable them to understand the gravity of any future pregnancy for all involved.

Moving forward, in the short term I would consider using 'google translate' or similar programme to write a note to Sasha; first, asking for her consent to discuss this issue with her at all, and then to ask whether she is happy for her daughter to be present.

I would arrange a meeting as soon as possible with both Sasha and her husband (given their agreement) and explain all the risks, including the husband's risk of losing both his wife and baby. It is important that the husband is fully informed. It may be that he has not considered the ripple effect that refusing to allow contraception may have on himself, his wife and his other children and what that could mean for him both psychologically and financially. He would be responsible for all his family care if Sasha was to lose her life through another pregnancy, and this would presumably hinder his ability to work and earn money.

I would also give Sasha the option of talking to a GP or surgeon confidentially, again with a translator present, which might increase the chance of a longer term solution such as undergoing a sterilisation, once she has recovered from her previous surgery.

DAVID'S REFLECTIONS ON THIS SCENARIO

This scenario is fairly sparsely presented so I need to fill in some gaps. However I do this, using **PSP** is a real challenge, requiring significant imagination and sensitivity. But I can try.

(Continued)

The persons involved are Sasha, the husband, the daughter and the midwife. In order to use **PSP** in any helpful way I have to ask these questions: Of the people involved, what influences does each bring with them? What are their goals at this moment? And this is not at all easy to say.

Sasha does not speak or read English so without involving her daughter it will be difficult or impossible to establish her wishes, and of course it may be that involving her daughter is not what she wants in any case.

I have the husband's view on hearsay, so all I can do is assume that this is a true report.

I can ask the daughter if she a) would tell me what her mother wants me to do and b) if she would be prepared to translate.

I can ask the midwife what she thinks.

But beyond this it is very hard even to imagine what it is like to be a woman in a culture where the husband decides everything – how does that feel?

All I can do is make assumptions:

1. Sasha is willing to be helped by health services since she has made appointments
2. The husband is ok with this and knows his wife is presently being seen without him
3. Sasha understands the risk of death, as explained by the surgeon
4. Sasha is at risk of a further pregnancy
5. The husband speaks English

I am not first analysing this situation using any of the tools and approaches in this book – not even the Ethical Grid – since it seems imperative to clarify as much as I can before intervening further. And to try to get a sense of what it is like for the people involved, and what their situations are. I want to create autonomy for Sasha and not to cause harm, but it really is not clear how to achieve this.

My intuition, such as it is, is to arrange an urgent – even emergency – appointment with the husband and wife so as to explain, or explain again – with an interpreter present – the very high risk of pregnancy and to see if the couple are prepared to be helped together. Since this is seen as a family matter in their culture I feel justified in trying to work with both of them.

So, I would try to use **PSP** as far as possible as I picture the situation, and also use the Ethical Grid in the end, as is suggested below. Using this method I would most likely choose the tiles:

Risk

Serve needs first

Minimise harm

Create autonomy (for the group – i.e. the family)

I could also try other approaches, but clearly each would quickly reach a point where their usefulness was exhausted.

So, I would work urgently with the husband and wife and not involve the daughter, because of the risks to her and the risks in general of my making matters worse.

I would see what happens and make my next judgement from that point.

SUGGESTION FOR SCENARIO 7.5: APPLY PSP TO THIS SCENARIO PLUS THE ETHICAL GRID

SCENARIO 7.6: SELF-HARM OR THERAPY?

CATEGORIES: RIGHTS, AUTONOMY, RISK

Sharon is 36 with mild to moderate learning disabilities. She lives in a group home where she is looked after by a multidisciplinary professional team.

Sharon has a long history of self-harming, dating back to when she was a teenager. She also has persistent underlying depression for which she is receiving treatment. She normally responds well to this treatment, but only so long as she is allowed to self-harm. Her self-harming mostly consists of scratching her arms and legs with her fingernails to the point of bleeding, interfering with healing by repeatedly picking at scabs, and occasionally pulling her hair to cause herself pain, which has led to some hair loss. Her self-harming is currently permitted for up to 15 minutes a day, supervised.

A new member of staff – Fadeswa – has recently joined the organisation. She is the same grade as you, but considerably younger. In team meetings she often disagrees with you, in fact you are beginning to think she does this on purpose.

Fadeswa has focused on Sharon's care and repeatedly voiced opposition to the policy of allowing her to self-harm. Instead, Fadeswa wants to restrain Sharon when unsupervised and to make sure that all means of self-harming are not available to her. She insists that restraint would protect all involved in her care.

What do you think? Would you agree to Fadeswa's idea?

Do you agree with the proposal below?

EXAMPLE PROPOSAL FOR FOCUS: It is proposed that Sharon should be restrained to prevent self-harming.

Source: Case originally created by Bernie Davis (Coventry University).

VANESSA'S REFLECTIONS ON THIS SCENARIO

Because in the absence of other means of therapeutic outlet, self-harming is merely a coping mechanism and intervention which allows feelings and emotions to be externalised, I would support continuing the present policy.

Stopping this lady from self-harming, with restraint will, in itself, potentially lead to feelings of increased frustration from having her free will and liberty suppressed.

This will only serve to reinforce any issues Sharon may be struggling with which have control (or the lack of it) at the root cause of her depression. Allowing self-harming, for a limited period, supervised and within a safe environment, I think is reasonable under the circumstances at present. Although alarming for those observing, it does not imply any suicidal intent nor does it mean she is necessarily placing others at risk.

If self-harming is therapeutic to her then it should be accepted as a short-term measure until a more acceptable therapeutic intervention and outlet for her can be explored and initiated. To do this, and not to restrain her, facilitates the opening up and exploration of her current difficulties, by means of therapeutic communication, in whatever form that takes.

DAVID'S REFLECTIONS ON THIS SCENARIO

It is hard to use **PSP** in Sharon's case because it is difficult for me to imagine wanting or needing to do this, though in a way I do a version of this myself, by exercising through pain and by using alcohol to help me relax.

Writing the above paragraph was spontaneous and it allowed me – perhaps – a small door into Sharon's situation. If her 'self-harming' makes her feel more in control or happier, and if that is what she wants to do, then it is understandable, though not particularly desirable, the way I look at the world.

Sharon is depressed and has learning difficulties and is dependent on health and social care. This is not a free and creative life and it must be extraordinarily frustrating for her. Through her eyes self-harm is a form of relief from an existence she did not ask for and is presently enduring.

If I were her health carer I would be focusing on meeting her basic needs in a less physically damaging way, and on helping her, if possible, to find a more creative purpose in her life. I assume the team in the home is already attempting to do this, but I would want to look at what they are doing and see if there are other possibilities to try.

As far as the direct ethical issue is concerned – using the **NMC Code** and the law in addition to **PSP** – I would need to research and carry out 'slow thinking'. As far as the **Code** is concerned, I would be more puzzled than anything else. For example, as a nurse I would be required to:

14.1 act immediately to put right the situation if someone has suffered actual harm for any reason or an incident has happened which had the potential for harm

17.1 take all reasonable steps to protect people who are vulnerable or at risk from harm, neglect or abuse

4.1 balance the need to act in the best interests of people at all times with the requirement to respect a person's right to accept or refuse treatment

2.5 respect, support and document a person's right to accept or refuse care and treatment

This would be rather confusing. It would be unclear to me at least if I am supposed to stop the actual harm (**14.1**) or respect Sharon's rights to 'treat herself', since self-harming does appear to be a form of therapy (**4.1**). I don't think the **Code** would help me, and I would therefore need to decide for myself, ideally in collaboration with colleagues and Sharon herself.

I am also unsure whether Fadeswa's idea to restrain Sharon when not supervised is legal or reasonable.

The Mental Health Act 1983 Code of Practice 2015 says:

Restrictive interventions are deliberate acts on the part of other person(s) that restrict a patient's movement, liberty and/or freedom to act independently in order to:

- Take immediate control of a dangerous situation where there is a real possibility of harm to the person or others if no action is undertaken,

and

- End or reduce significantly the danger to the patient or others.
- Restrictive interventions should not be used to punish or for the sole intention of inflicting pain, suffering or humiliation. (**152**)

However, it is not clear how 'dangerous' the self-harming is (is it sufficiently dangerous to legally mandate restraint?). The team would need to take legal advice if restraint is being seriously considered.

My thinking – both 'fast' and 'slow' – is that if this is what Sharon chooses to do, and it is not harming other people, and we can work with her to see if she wants to change, then she should not only be allowed to continue self-harm but to be supported in this, and not be negatively judged.

SUGGESTION FOR SCENARIO 7.6: APPLY PSP TO THIS SCENARIO PLUS THE NMC CODE AND THE LAW

—— SCENARIO 7.7: SAVING MARJA? ——

CATEGORIES: RIGHTS, LAW, INFORMED CONSENT

Marja, a 34-year-old woman, who emigrated from Macedonia three years ago, has been admitted to your unit for a procedure to replace a faulty breast implant, under general anaesthetic. Marja has no family in this country and presently is not in a relationship.

During the pre-op period, the surgeon, Mr Rees, visited Marja to examine her and obtain consent for the replacement of the implant. During the examination, Mr Rees could clearly feel lumps under the axillary area (Marja's armpit) but did not say anything at the time, although his observations were documented in the clinical notes. However, he did not verbally mention the lumps to the attending nurse chaperoning during the examination.

During the operation, Mr Rees decided to look a little closer at the palpable lumps and went on to remove them surgically in order to send them to the lab. Marja was told of this after the procedure and was sent for at an outpatients appointment, during which Mr Rees informed her that she had a diagnosis of breast cancer, which had been confirmed by pathology on the removed lumps.

Marja was devastated by this news and became angry and upset that the surgeon had removed the lumps without informed consent from her.

You are the nurse attending Marja at the Clinic. She is very upset and finds it hard to voice her objections since English is not her first language. You are aware that the law clearly states that informed consent must be sought and given to surgery in non-emergency situations. You are also aware that it might be possible for Marja to sue Mr Rees for negligence leading to trespass.

How should you advise Marja? Do you agree with the proposal below?

EXAMPLE PROPOSAL FOR FOCUS: It is proposed that you should advise Marja that she could sue the surgeon for negligence leading to trespass.

VANESSA'S REFLECTIONS ON THIS SCENARIO

In my opinion there is a clear case here of professional and legal negligence leading to trespass. I have the following reasons:

1) There was a duty of care to inform Marja of proposed surgery, risks, benefits and alternatives. This standard was obviously breached by the surgeon.
2) Although the surgeon's actions were benevolent and were carried out in what he believed to be in Marja's best interests, the surgeon failed to inform her or gain consent. This was in my opinion unreasonable, and led to psychological and physical harm, which was foreseeable.

Even though Marja would more than likely have given consent to have the lumps from her breast removed, she still should have been informed kindly and sensitively by the surgeon that lumps were found at the pre-op examination, and had the options explained to her. Clinical professionals have a legal duty to obtain informed consent from every patient, and Marja had the capacity to make her own decisions regarding her own health.

Although legally I think Marja would have a valid and actionable claim for negligence against this surgeon, I think (speaking from personal experience of pursuing a litigation claim) that to sue in this instance could end up being potentially counterproductive for her. This action could lead to a long drawn-out process, which might result in more psychological trauma for her unless the hospital Trust (who are responsible vicariously) and the surgeon involved were quick to admit liability, and settle the claim swiftly, which is rarely the case in today's ethos.

Having said all of that, I strongly believe that it is entirely up to Marja about how she would like to proceed from here and would understand her reasons for pursuing either option.

I also think that the surgeon, in the interests of candour, should apologise to Marja at the earliest opportunity and explain his reasoning for his omission. With the right timely support, honesty and care, I think that Marja may regain the trust that has been lost, though a lot also depends on health professionals being honest and keeping her properly informed throughout her care and treatment in future. A sad result of this omission is that she is bound to always wonder if she is being told the truth in the future, which will affect her capacity to deal with her treatment and recovery in a beneficial way.

DAVID'S REFLECTIONS ON THIS SCENARIO

I feel a lot of sympathy for Marja and, personally, I find the surgeon's disregard for her autonomy and legal entitlement outrageous. I can certainly imagine how scared and alienated Marja would be feeling, not least without close support in her country of residence.

I would not want to project my feelings of anger on to Marja, and would check out with her exactly how she is feeling. I would certainly want to explore the option of

(Continued)

counselling and to find her group support for her cancer treatment, and to encourage her autonomy in any other way I could, by assisting with basic needs, the provision of information, education and to help her feel less alone.

If I were her and this had happened to me I would strongly consider suing the surgeon, not least so that he was not so careless in future. So, I would set out the matter to her as I see it, and I would tell her what I would do, I would say 'this is how I see the situation'. I would of course caution her about the risks, but I would say that if she feels strongly after a time of contemplation – a cooling-off period – then she should, if she wishes, and with my support and that of an interpreter, talk to Mr Rees (if he will talk to her) and if she is still not satisfied she should commence legal action against him.

SUGGESTION FOR SCENARIO 7.7: APPLY PSP TO THIS SCENARIO PLUS THE LAW AND RISK ANALYSIS

— SCENARIO 7.8: SAFETY IN SECLUSION? —

CATEGORIES: MENTAL HEALTH, LAW, PATIENT RIGHTS, RESOURCES

Tom is a 45-year-old man who's been in a high-level secure mental health unit for the past ten years, due to repeated offending.

Tom has a diagnosis of Paranoid Schizophrenia. Medication and therapeutic approaches have failed to reduce his delusions and paranoia, and he continues to have frequent violent and aggressive outbursts against certain members of staff. Tom spends some of his time in seclusion in order, it is claimed, to prevent the risk of harm to others.

Tom explains that he feels aggressive when he hears loud voices or when others prolong their eye contact with him, which he finds intimidating. He also becomes very withdrawn and depressed when he's in seclusion, will often resort to head-banging as a protest, and mostly refuses to eat or drink when he finds himself in this situation. As a result, Tom has lost a considerable amount of weight over the last six months.

You're a care worker on this busy, short-staffed secure unit. You've noticed that when a certain member of staff is on duty Tom tends to be put into seclusion more often, which seems to have the effect of making him more aggressive. This member of staff, Tony, a Registered Mental Health Nurse, who qualified six months ago, is regularly put in charge of the shift. Tony has a loud authoritative voice and is often seen 'squaring up' to Tom, maintaining eye contact with him when he feels Tom's 'about to kick off'. This appears to provoke Tom to lash out at Tony. The usual result is that Tom's put into seclusion for the rest of the shift to 'protect the staff and patients from potential or actual harm'. Tony 'doesn't have time for Tom's games' and argues that his strategy 'frees up our time to take care of the other high dependency patients'.

What do you think is appropriate in this situation?

EXAMPLE PROPOSAL FOR FOCUS: It is proposed that it is appropriate to place Tom into seclusion when he lashes out physically at Tony.

VANESSA'S REFLECTIONS ON THIS SCENARIO

This is a reflection provided by an anonymous healthcare worker who responded to this issue on the Values Exchange, after I posted it as part of an ethics education programme. He tells me that he works on a forensics unit just like the one presented, and has experienced this scenario or variations of it many times.

I have included his response (verbatim) here as I feel he has applied **PSP** without even being aware of it, as many of us do all the time. I feel it demonstrates many elements of **PSP**, including personal knowledge, experience and perceptions, awareness of others and plans for action.

PSP is not a formal approach, and may seem vague at times. But we find it a powerful reminder of the variety of human experience even where the circumstances are shared, and we believe it should be at the forefront of consciousness all the time: which persons are involved? What do they personally bring to the circumstances? How do they see the circumstances? How does the relationship between them and the circumstances create different situations? Can these situations be conveyed to others? What plan can we make, and how does this fit with the purpose of health care?

All these aspects can be identified in the voice of this health professional, even though they are not explicitly stated:

There are a number of issues around this scenario and it's not as simple as using seclusion for convenience.

The first thing I would ask is has there been any type of independent mediation between Tom and Tony? If not, why not? Tony could explain, in a settled controlled environment his actions and Tom could also reiterate his feelings.

Next you have to consider other patients. With the information to hand it appears to be a busy short-staffed ward. These other patients have needs to be met also. If you are using limited existing ward resources to manage Tom on a shift-by-shift basis then other patients will not be getting the treatment and care they deserve because of Tom, this could create an issue for Tom's safety if this is identified by his peer group, which in my experience, would happen.

(Continued)

Third, if mediation and discussion made zero inroads over a period of time, it may be better to move Tony from the ward, see Tom's reaction and then review it after a three-month period. It may be that Tony starts to target someone else, again a regular scenario which has happened on many occasions.

Finally, if the ward is short staffed, why isn't it being supported, why aren't issues raised through IR1s, management and H&S reps, both union and management appointed?

The factors that can trigger Tom's aggressive behaviour are already known to staff; I believe Tony's staring at him as a warning is passive aggressive and antagonises the situation. The whole situation could be avoided with a few minutes helping Tom out, in the long run this would be better to prevent Tom self-harming when put in seclusion. This situation can upset other patients as well. I would speak to a Manager and explain I don't want to get Tony into trouble but I feel he is making the situation worse for the unit as a whole, Tom deserves as much respect as other patients and regardless of Tony's personal views he should treat him the same as others. Finding ways of working with people is always better in my opinion!

I feel that seclusion should be used as a last resort and not as a normality. The root causes of Tom's behaviour should be looked into and a resolution found. Tony is obviously part of this root cause and mediation between the two should be instigated as a matter of urgency to stop the situation getting further out of hand.

It is not in Tom's best interest to be put in seclusion, this makes him self-harm and not eat properly. Tony should know the triggers that cause Tom to lash out and should do his best to avoid these instead of trying to give him a 'warning' look. The team should come up with a care plan to try to help Tom as that is what the staff are there for, to meet the needs of all the patients. I would have to speak to the manager about what I have seen Tony doing as this is extremely unfair to Tom.

We both applaud this health carer and are proud to offer his thoughts as an example of compassionate, practical healthcare.

DAVID'S REFLECTIONS ON THIS SCENARIO

Mental healthcare is a minefield of conceptual confusion and practical challenges and, as a result, can often leave people like Tom in a horrible limbo where nothing is being done to help them live a meaningful life.

There is little detail in the scenario, so I would have questions:

1. Is Tom guilty of a crime? Is he imprisoned under sentence?
2. Is Tom mentally ill, and is he 'sectioned' – made to be in the unit in the best interests of himself and others?

These questions are central, in several ways, not least to the way Tom sees himself and others see him.

As it stands, his status is unclear. He is obviously unhappy and does not want to be on the unit so presumably he is forced to be there, either as a patient or a criminal or both. And if he is a patient then he is facing the prospect of unlimited detention, in a place where he very clearly does not want to be, and is not helping him.

In any event, the fact that he does not want to be there at least gives us some indication of how he sees the situation.

3. What is the purpose of his seclusion – is it to protect him or others or both?

This is another central question, not least with regard to the **plan** part of **PSP** – if his seclusion is to benefit others more than Tom this will have a radical effect on any plan, and on how Tom and others see their situations. If it is to benefit Tom then how it offers benefit needs to be explained.

Other questions that spring to mind are:

4. If 'mental healthcare' cannot help Tom, what mental illness does he have?

Tom has been in the unit for ten years, and he does not seem to be improving. Why is this? What sickness does he have, what treatments has he had, and why have they not helped?

5. With regard to the seclusion, if it is both to help Tom and protect others, what other ways to manage things have been tried to do this?
6. Is seclusion a punishment or a therapy?

Whatever it is – punishment, therapy or both – what is the evidence that it will work to achieve whatever end it is intended to achieve?

To me, the **person** part of **PSP** is also vital here. From the scenario it appears that Tom and Tony have an antagonistic relationship, and that Tony possibly enjoys enforcing his will over Tom. Does Tony deliberately provoke Tom, for some reason?

It is possible that Tom's and Tony's perceptions are extremely different – as are their social positions. Tom may see Tony as his gaoler – which he effectively is – and Tony may see Tom as a 'bad person' or a problem that must be controlled, for whatever mix of reasons. Does Tony get pleasure from secluding Tom? Does Tom's mental health become worse as a consequence of repeated seclusions? Does Tom fear Tony? Do they both see themselves as enemies?

(Continued)

Whatever the case, this is not a happy set of circumstances, and it is hard to see how it can be described as 'work for health'. It seems that nothing is being done therapeutically for Tom, and that the only goal of the staff, certainly of Tony, is to get Tom off the main ward rather than help him.

However, I do see a role for **PSP** here. I think that there should be facilitated meetings between Tom and Tony – and others if this is felt to be helpful – and that these meetings should be designed for Tom and Tony to see each other as **persons**, with life histories, hopes and vulnerabilities. Both Tom and Tony should be supported to explain their present **situations** – to describe the world as they see and experience it. By doing this it may help Tony understand Tom's illness experiences – the intrusive voices, for example – and how this makes him feel intimidated, anxious and depressed. It may help Tony see Tom as a person, and vice versa.

There is presently such a difference in their situations that an intervention is necessary, for Tom's health and for Tony's sensitivity and understanding of his purpose.

So, no, I do not think further seclusion should be carried out and a calming intervention, such as described above, should be undertaken immediately.

I also feel that after ten years Tom's entire care programme must be reviewed and if it is failing then it needs to be changed, with Tom's full involvement.

SUGGESTION FOR SCENARIO 7.8: APPLY PSP TO THIS SCENARIO PLUS THE ETHICAL GRID AND THE LAW

—— SCENARIO 7.9: TERMINAL JEOPARDY ——

CATEGORIES: ONCOLOGY, CHOICE, AUTONOMY, CONSENT

You're a registered health professional working on an Oncology ward. You're caring for a group of patients who have cancer in varying degrees of severity.

One of your patients, Janet, has end-stage lung cancer and is presently struggling to breathe. She has malignant pleural effusion, which has now stopped responding to usual pleurodesis drainage efforts. Fluid accumulation is recurring rapidly and causing shortness of breath. Because of bone metastases Janet's also suffering from severe pain in her back and chest area.

Janet is now profoundly fatigued from her continued respiratory effort and disease effect, and has become agitated and restless. Her gathered family are clearly distressed by Janet's obvious and extreme suffering.

Your senior nurse discusses administering another dose of Diamorphine to Janet, which has already been prescribed. However, if you do administer the extra dose it's likely, though not certain, that Janet will go into respiratory depression and ultimately stop breathing.

What would you do in this situation and how would you feel about it? Do you agree with the proposal below?

EXAMPLE PROPOSAL FOR FOCUS: It is proposed that you administer another dose of Diamorphine to Janet.

VANESSA'S REFLECTIONS ON THIS SCENARIO

I would explain the benefit vs risk and alternatives in what I see essentially as a 'double effect' scenario, I would gain consent from the patient assuming capacity and take an enabling role to assist her to understand and discuss with the family their wishes also. But ultimately, if this is what the patient requires and requests, then my intent would be to eliminate the ACTUAL pain rather than focus on the POTENTIAL problem which may come from it. This would also have to be done in a timely manner, and a discussion with the family may not even be possible without Janet suffering pain for a longer period of time.

The act of giving Diamorphine to relieve pain is benevolent. It is to will the positive effect only, not the death of the patient. My act would be carried out for the primary reason of responding to actual need. I would give the pain relief as soon as possible.

Yes, this patient's respiratory centre might be further depressed by giving additional Diamorphine, and this could potentially be reversed with a dose of Naloxone, for example, if respiratory rate dropped to a certain defined level, though I would see this intervention as futile. It might also result once again in her being in a position where her pain is unmanaged. In my view, more harm could arise for her, both psychologically and physiologically, from the effects of being in constant, and well-established pain than if we take the risk.

DAVID'S REFLECTIONS ON THIS SCENARIO

I would clearly, calmly and gently explain the risks and the likely effect of the additional Diamorphine to Janet, if I could, and suggest that she discusses this with her family, since they are present.

(Continued)

Janet is terminally ill and is aware of this and, despite the severe pain, she does appear to have decision-making capacity. The injection will offer her some pain-relief and perhaps a little peace, so if she were to say she would like the injection, I would have no hesitation in giving it to her.

Thinking of **PSP** I am very aware that this is a personal judgement, in part influenced by my own views about the value of human life in an unimaginably huge universe.

SUGGESTION FOR SCENARIO 7.9: APPLY PSP TO THIS SCENARIO PLUS COST—BENEFIT ANALYSIS

— SCENARIO 7.10: ADVOCATE FOR WHOM? —

CATEGORIES: ONCOLOGY, CHOICE, AUTONOMY, CONSENT

Three months ago, Sam (39) was diagnosed with an aggressive brain tumour. He has a Glioblastoma in the frontal lobe of his brain. Sam is currently expected to live for approximately another 12–18 months maximum, even with treatment, although this could be shorter if his tumour re-grows suddenly or a new tumour appears.

Sam was initially diagnosed after presenting to his GP with focal seizures, headaches, nausea and vomiting, irritability and mood swings. Due to the nature and location of Sam's Grade IV tumour, he's only received surgery for a diagnostic biopsy, to debulk the tumour mass (which is complex) and to reduce intracranial pressure (ICP) arising from the tumour.

Sam has had radiotherapy and adjuvant IV chemotherapy following surgery. He is now nearing the end of a course of oral chemotherapy to attempt to suppress re-growth and extend his life. Sam also takes prophylactic anticonvulsant drugs, and his seizures are currently well managed.

Sam has been prescribed antidepressants and is also taking steroids (Dexamethasone) to reduce inflammation and the effects of ICP from his disease.

Following a fall at home Sam has been admitted to the palliative care unit where you work. Sam's wife (Angela) reports that he fell while attempting to get out of bed in the middle of the night, and seemed confused when she talked to him. Sam was not physically injured in the fall.

Doctors discovered a chest infection on admission, which they suspect may have caused the confusion. The infection itself was probably caused by low white cell counts, which are one consequence of chemotherapy treatment. Following two days of appropriate antibiotic therapy Sam's blood cell counts have recovered well, and he's now improved significantly.

Sam currently appears to have capacity once reasonable adjustments are made to aid him in communications. At most times during the day he's clear and lucid and able to make decisions. Sam has a delay in processing information due to his illness, and needs longer to think and respond in conversation. He's less likely to be lucid at night-time, when he is lying down, which is thought to be due to raised ICP from the effects of staying in this position for extended periods.

Sam can feed himself and wash his upper body parts, but needs assistance with standing, due to poor muscle control and spasms. He suffers with poor co-ordination when walking and has dizzy spells. Sam is assessed as a falls risk.

Sam and Angela live in an adapted bungalow, which they moved into a month ago, once they knew Sam's prognosis. They have no children, and no close relatives living nearby. Angela is currently not working, in order to care for Sam. Sam says Angela often becomes stressed about her situation as main carer and sometimes takes it out on him verbally, when she's feeling low.

Sam was formerly an engineer for a telecommunications company, and has also had to give up work due to his illness and its effects, which he finds enormously frustrating. He's also had to give up his passion for bike riding, which he previously used for exercise and stress relief. Sam is currently receiving disability benefits to help with his care and to help with the couple's mounting financial burdens.

Currently, home assistance comprises of shower/toileting support once daily, in the mornings, for 30 minutes. This help is provided free, by social services. Sam also receives a weekly visit from the community nursing team for medications management issues such as pain relief/seizure control, which are currently well managed. Sam is also in touch with the Neurology Specialist Nurse, who visits once monthly. She is expected to be more involved once Sam's disease shows evidence of re-growth and deterioration, and radiotherapy and chemotherapy have been stopped. An end of life plan has been set up which states that, if possible, Sam should be cared for at home, as this is his expressed wish. Support will come from the Macmillan team and will be co-ordinated by the Neurology Specialist Nurse.

Angela says that despite daily home assistance services she can't watch Sam constantly and so simply can't care for him at home anymore – in fact she's 'at the end of her tether'. Angela is concerned that Sam is already showing signs of deterioration and is frightened that things will now worsen quickly. However, recent tests have shown no advance in the tumour. Nevertheless, Angela remains resolute that she can no longer care for Sam and his immediate needs full-time – and wishes to return to work as a legal secretary part-time.

Sam is aware of his wife's concerns and needs but is equally adamant – and very clearly states – that he wants to go home: he is feeling better, and he asks for your help.

Who, if anyone, should you advocate for? Do you agree with the proposal below?

EXAMPLE PROPOSAL FOR FOCUS: It is proposed that you advocate for Sam and assist him to discharge back to his own home.

(153, 154, 155, 156, 157)

VANESSA'S REFLECTIONS ON THIS SCENARIO

This scenario mainly involves mainly Sam and Angela. It's complex, but I would advocate for Sam to go home, after working to support the couple.

From Sam's point of view, he is seriously ill and wants to be cared for at home, with his wife by his side, and this is also reflected in his End of Life plan (**EoL**). He also says he's feeling better and appears less confused now that his chest infection has been treated. Sam may not realise why his wife has suddenly decided she can't care for him any more and may be feeling angry and rejected, or he may feel that he's a burden to Angela: so the issue needs to be addressed urgently with him, both with and without Angela present.

From Angela's point of view, the situation is different. Though there is little information about Angela, some reasonable assumptions can be made. During my career I experienced this type of behaviour from a loved one (caring in an adapted home for her husband who was suffering a severe debilitating neurological condition). If we can understand her point of view better then we can help both of them get to a place where they feel supported and both have their needs met as much as possible. For this reason, my main focus would be upon Angela in this scenario.

I can imagine that Angela feels very tired, scared and lonely. She may well miss parts of Sam that she once knew, and she may miss physical contact and intimacy. She is likely to feel that she has no control, and is unheard and unsupported. She may be feeling inadequate in meeting her husband's needs and fearful of what the future may look like for both her and Sam as his disease progresses.

Despite Angela's earlier wish to have an adapted home, it's not unusual for carers – especially family carers – to quickly feel burnt out both emotionally and physically from caring for a loved one who's become so dependent. The toll an illness like Sam's takes from them can be truly heavy.

In these situations, the main carer can sometimes become resentful because they have little time to do things of their own, such as meeting friends or just having some alone or down time on a daily basis. These feelings can make a carer feel guilty and tend not to be verbalised. I have witnessed a close family carer start snapping at the dependent person and lose patience when these issues for the carer are not addressed.

Moving forward I think there should be a multidisciplinary team meeting, which Angela and Sam should also attend. The meeting should consider what further support could be offered to Angela, including how to reduce the risk of falls, to explore Angela and Sam's feelings, and to find a way forward with which everyone agrees. There are options for compromise – such as offering respite care for Sam – to enable Angela to have a regular break and something to look forward to without feeling guilty. Angela and Sam could also receive therapy sessions, either separately or as a couple, to help them verbalise their emotions and move forward in a positive way, which will prevent resentment building up.

The specialist nurse could also be involved in assisting and reassuring Angela that Sam is not yet at the point where he is approaching **EoL** care. And there are peer support groups that Angela and Sam could join, as well as online fora. If they can both appreciate each other's **situations** – the **S** in **PSP** – this will allow them to be more patient and understanding of each other, which is essential if a therapeutic liaison is to continue between them, and Sam is to get the care he needs as his disease progresses further.

DAVID'S REFLECTIONS ON THIS SCENARIO

This is a good case on which to use **PSP**, since we know quite a bit about Sam and something about Angela. There is something of a mystery as to why – having moved into a specially adapted bungalow only a month ago, and giving up work to care for her husband – Angela no longer wishes to help Sam with his fundamental need to be cared for at home, especially as his primary condition does not appear to have changed since that decision. Though of course the reality of full-time care would hit home quickly once it starts and Angela may well now feel the decision was a mistake.

As far as **PSP** is concerned, we have a good idea of the first **P (person)** as it relates to Sam, but less idea where Angela is concerned. The same applies to the **S (situation)** – we know Sam's **situation** – he is ill and desperately wants to stay at home, that seems to be all that matters to him at this late stage of his life. But Angela's **situation** is not clear. Why has she changed her mind from only one month earlier?

Looking at the proposal, and considering the Ethical Grid as suggested below, I do not see this as a matter of advocating for Sam. I see the need for a more creative and sensitive solution, that tries to bring the couple together in a united second **P** – a joint **plan.**

The big question, from the Grid, is for whom are you working? Are you trying to enable one individual or two, and if it is two, are you trying to support them singly and separately, or as a couple? This is very obviously a matter of personal judgement.

Using **PSP** it is clearly important to find out how Angela is feeling, what she wants and needs, how she sees the situation as it is and as it might be in the future. Since she is saying she cannot cope, is frightened and sees the situation as already deteriorated so much that Sam needs residential care, it is essential to talk to her immediately in order to clarify, and to calmly look at the circumstances together – are they really so bad that her husband cannot return home? How does she feel about how he feels? How does she feel about their relationship? Are they a couple still?

(Continued)

I think too, once you can see the situation as Angela sees it, you should meet with the couple and look at what extra practical support Angela would need to have Sam home, if she is prepared to support him in that. If she isn't, then I think work for health would have to be undertaken to Sam and Angela separately, but for now we should look to creating autonomy for them as a couple.

I do think that counselling for the couple should be tried too, so they can freely express their fears and wishes openly to one another – so that they can both appreciate the situation as the other sees it.

You also need to deal with Sam's request. He wants to go home and appears to be capable of supporting himself there with assistance, despite being a falls risk. Given this, I believe that you must work for his health by meeting as many of his basic needs as possible, and by making it as easy as possible for him to return home. It will then be up to Sam and Angela to work out – one way or another – how they will deal with his imminent return.

SUGGESTION FOR SCENARIO 7.10: APPLY PSP TO THIS SCENARIO PLUS THE ETHICAL GRID

SCENARIO 7.11: COMPULSORY MEDICATION TO SILENCE THE VOICES?

CATEGORIES: PSYCHIATRY, FORENSICS, LAW, MENTAL HEALTH

Peter, a 26-year-old black British man, has a generally happy life with his partner – Lucy, who is a white British woman – and his three young children. However, he recently assaulted a passer-by in the street where he lives.

Peter claims that this person – a young man of Asian descent – said something racist to him. When interviewed by police, the victim stated firmly that he did not speak to Peter. Lucy, who was walking with Peter at the time, claims to have heard nothing.

When encouraged to talk about Peter, Lucy says she's noticed his personal hygiene has declined recently, and he seems to have become more 'distracted', which has caused her to become increasingly concerned about their relationship.

The police referred Peter to mental health services. After a period of initial assessment he's now been admitted to a low secure unit under section 37 of the Mental Health Act (1983) (**138**) with a diagnosis of Schizophrenia.

Current assessments seem to indicate that Peter is a serious risk to himself and others, particularly in response to auditory hallucinations which tell him he's wicked.

Peter has so far declined any medication, citing evidence from a recent research paper that suggests that antipsychotics are over-prescribed for black people. Peter also has expressed concern that the proposed medication will affect his ability to concentrate on his Open University Psychology course, which he intends to continue, whether or not he's an inpatient.

Most of the clinical team are of the view that without antipsychotic medication Peter's distress is likely to escalate. They also believe that if Peter were well, he would not be a risk. The consultant in charge of his care proposes that they seek a second opinion from an appointed doctor, and that, if everyone agrees, Peter should be given antipsychotic medication against his will under section 58 of the Mental Health Act.

Whenever you speak with Peter, he does appear a little distracted, but calm and lucid when answering questions and justifying his reasoning. He does admit to hearing frequent voices of a malevolent nature, but says he can deal with this. He argues that he is well enough to have treatment in the community but will stay on the ward if that is what is required. However, he is very clear that he does not want this medication.

What would you do in this scenario? Do you agree with the proposal below?

EXAMPLE PROPOSAL FOR FOCUS: It is proposed that you support Peter in his refusal to accept medication.

VANESSA'S REFLECTIONS ON THIS SCENARIO

I can't really say anything that hasn't already been said by David in his comprehensive reflection below. I agree totally with his view on this. The only difference is personal – though we may agree about what is right we all bring different interpretations to any circumstances.

My own motivation comes strongly from a position where a person close to me was diagnosed with this schizophrenia during my early nursing career. This person, who was very dear to me, was given antipsychotics against his will under a section order.

It was distressing to witness the psychological suffering, which arose both from the acute psychosis and equally from the forceful detainment and administration of these powerful drugs. The side-effects for this person were highly disabling also. It's difficult – probably impossible – for me to stand away from this scenario and not be influenced by my personal experience. I learnt a lot and formed strong opinions about how persons with mental health are treated and how their liberty and dignity can be eroded. It now seems so obvious to me that empowering these persons should be the first step in safeguarding them.

If I were working in this field now I would consider it imperative to try different and less damaging therapeutic interventions, such as 'talking therapy'.

DAVID'S REFLECTIONS ON THIS SCENARIO

In this case I would focus on the first **P** – Peter, the **person**, and try to understand what drives him and how he sees the world. I would also carefully consider my own motivations and biases, on a continuing basis.

Three things are clear: 1) Peter does not want medication that will muddy his thinking, even though he hears malevolent voices; 2) the clinicians agree that he should have the medication; and 3) they are legally entitled to administer it to Peter against his wishes, in his 'best interests'. What is not clear is what impact the medication will have – it may help Peter or it may harm him, or it may have little impact (though forcing it upon him against his wishes is likely to upset him, as it would most people).

My personal feeling, informed by years of research, writing and teaching in mental health contexts, is that since Peter is lucid and will accept help so long as it does not involve medication, then his wishes should be respected. There are many therapies that do not involve medication that could and should be tried (**158**). There are also well-known arguments that 'mental illness' is a social construct rather than a reality, and that we should all accept responsibility for our actions, and be encouraged to do so (**159, 160**).

Self-awareness is of central importance for me, in this case. I have worked in several psychiatric environments and observed practices and justifications from staff with which I profoundly disagree. I have even appeared at Mental Health Tribunals on behalf of patients trapped in the system, giving evidence against the psychiatrists, and I have spoken at several 'psychiatric survivor' gatherings. And, from a philosophical point of view, I find much lacking in accepted concepts of 'mental illness', including the categorisations offered in various **DSMs** (**161**). Furthermore, my long-held theory of health leans heavily towards creating and respecting autonomy, and treating people equally. In short – I am massively and permanently biased.

I have to factor this in. My judgements – like everyone else's – do not leap into being from a vacuum – and I would want to make this clear to all involved: it may even be that I should withdraw from this matter, in case my presence and biases make things even worse for Peter.

But all this said, I believe what I believe, even though I am prejudiced (just as the clinicians are differently prejudiced) and I would, passionately, act on those beliefs and therefore do my utmost to support Peter in a journey to deal with his voices, and improve his life in ways he is comfortable with, which are effective, and which respect him as a unique person.

So, as I have done several times in the past, I would support the person, even against my colleagues, and would hope to do this in a respectful, professional and compassionate manner.

SUGGESTION FOR SCENARIO 7.11: APPLY PSP TO THIS SCENARIO PLUS THE ETHICAL GRID AND THE LAW

(162, 136)

—— SCENARIO 7.12: A TRICKY AFFAIR ——

CATEGORIES: CONSENT, CONFIDENTIALITY, FAMILY RELATIONSHIPS

John, a 55-year-old male, is in your care. He's developed bad chest pain, which he tells you feels like a very severe episode of angina, from which he's suffered for the last 18 months. His wife has accompanied John to your department and is obviously extremely concerned for her husband's health. She repeatedly tells you John's suffered a previous myocardial infarction (a heart attack) a few months ago. You've contacted the ambulance service, who are on their way, but may be up to 30 minutes.

As John's wife leaves to make a phone call to organise childcare, John asks if you would please keep his wife away while he makes a phone call of his own. Urgently he tries to dial, but nothing happens. Obviously agitated, he tries several more times, but cannot get a signal. He throws the phone to the floor and breaks down in tears.

You naturally ask him what's wrong. He shakes his head, says he feels so bad, then he tells you that he's been having an affair with a woman named Helen for the past five years. Helen knows he's married with two teenage children. She is also aware that John's family have no knowledge of the affair. Anxious for his health, John's desperate to see Helen. He hands you a card with her number on, and asks you to contact her to let her know he wants her to come in; she lives only a few minutes away. He says, 'of course I trust you won't say a word to my wife' and strongly impresses on you his desire that no one else whatsoever should be told of the situation.

John is very distressed and you are concerned about the effect of the situation on his health.

What should you do? Do you agree with the proposal below?

EXAMPLE PROPOSAL FOR FOCUS: It is proposed that you should do what John asks of you.

VANESSA'S REFLECTIONS ON THIS SCENARIO

This would be an uncomfortable situation for anyone to be in.

In this scenario my feelings of not wishing to deceive John's wife, who is obviously concerned for her husband, conflict with John's choice. John is asking

(Continued)

me to do something that I would feel very uncomfortable with (distracting his wife while he speaks and meets with his mistress, Helen). I consider that my first duty is to John and his immediate need to remain as calm as possible until the ambulance arrives.

John needs emergency treatment for a life-threatening condition. Any further anxiety is clearly not in his best interests, as this could increase his blood pressure and have a detrimental effect on his cardiac function. I imagine that his request is a difficult thing to ask you to do, and that he may well be feeling ashamed. And the risk and fear of his wife finding out about his concealed affair must also be uppermost in his mind at this worrying time.

We can assume that John's wife has no idea what is going on in the background and would most likely be devastated if she knew. I would imagine she would also be very cross and feel a deep sense of betrayal and further loss of trust if she found out that the health professional treating John was also concealing the truth.

I can imagine that if Helen has been in a relationship with John for five years then she would want to know what is happening with him. It seems reasonable to assume that they both have deep feelings for each other, this being a long-term affair. Helen would also be concerned about John's wife finding out about their relationship.

In conscience, the best I could do is offer the use of my own phone so he could talk with Helen, if he is able to. I might be willing to briefly inform her as a close friend to him, if he were not able to speak, although I wouldn't feel comfortable doing this if I'm honest. I would prefer him to speak with her directly if possible. Doing anything beyond this, I feel, would be acting deceptively.

I cannot refuse his right to talk to Helen and wouldn't necessarily want to. If he chooses to have an affair it is none of my business. I would also have a legal duty to uphold his confidence as what he has disclosed is not a safeguarding issue, does not involve a crime, and disclosure of this information is not in the wider public interest.

It is his right to have an affair, but it is also my right not to be complicit in the act, as this is not within my role and responsibilities, and may cause problems down the line.

DAVID'S REFLECTIONS ON THIS SCENARIO

This is an interesting example, and it seems right to use and examine intuition when addressing it.

My 'fast thinking' reaction was, instantly, 'no'. When I had this thought I was unclear why I chose 'no', and I remain unsure even on reflection – but it was a powerful rejection. I think I felt a mixture of being used, a sense that this is not my job, and confusion about whether I should get involved in any way with this, since it could easily turn out to cause considerable hurt to many people, and I don't want to hurt people if I can avoid it.

However, after only a few moments, these thoughts seemed to fall away – again I don't know why. For some reason, the request came to seem reasonable – Helen has been John's lover and friend for five years, so she is no different from any other close friend or relative that a patient has asked me to contact. Whatever I think of the context is irrelevant – or at least this is how I quickly came to see it.

So, I would do as he asks, in a simple and professional manner, and then carry on with the rest of my work, i.e.: 'We have a patient (giving his name) who has asked me to inform you that he is in the hospital at present, and has asked to see you.' I would not give any further information other than to explain where and when she could visit.

SUGGESTION FOR SCENARIO 7.12: APPLY PSP TO THIS SCENARIO PLUS INTUITION

— SCENARIO 7.13: COMPASSION FOR ALL? —

CATEGORIES: EMOTIONS, PROFESSIONAL ROLE, COMPASSION

Lucy is a 22-year-old nurse working on the neurology ward. She's an emotional person with an overt, compassionate nature. Lucy loves helping people, and she makes a point of comforting them in bad moments.

Today, a 41-year-old man, Phillip Smith, is brought to the ward accompanied by a policeman, to hear about some test results. He's a known and convicted criminal, who committed sexual assaults on five young teenagers ten years ago, and was convicted and imprisoned locally. Phillip is now on conditional release as part of his rehabilitation.

The test results show he has Motor Neurone Disease, which is a condition that leads to muscle weakness, often with visible wasting. It is an incurable, gradual disease. Anyone affected will, eventually, completely lose the ability to walk, talk and move, as the disease progresses.

The specialist neurologist asks Lucy to accompany him as he delivers the bad news to Phillip.

As the news sinks in Phillip becomes so distressed that he starts to cry in despair.

He looks at Lucy, and with his body language he asks her to support him. He clearly needs somebody to be with him in this terrible moment, if only to sit with him and hold his hand.

What should Lucy do? Do you agree with the proposal below?

EXAMPLE PROPOSAL FOR FOCUS: It is proposed that Lucy shows empathy, ignores his past and tries to help Phillip.

VANESSA'S REFLECTIONS ON THIS SCENARIO

This is a very difficult situation for any nurse to encounter. I think that although this was a very tragic incident that happened, and this man was clearly implicated in this, we have to make sure that we show compassion to all patients, no matter what their past is. This doesn't mean that you necessarily have to feel empathy for him. It just means that you are able to recognise that this is an emotional touch point for this patient and we have a legal, ethical and professional duty to respond appropriately. However, this does not mean that you are required to be a robot and your feelings around this issue are very important.

It is easy to make assumptions; for example, although this is not an excuse, and by no means condones his actions, we don't know whether this man was perhaps suffering from some form of psychosis, diminishing his responsibility somewhat, when he initiated the sexual assaults. This essentially means that he may have been severely mentally ill and may have lost capacity. He may have heard voices compelling him and threatening him, which are very real to him.

When cases like this arise, it is very important to seek clinical supervision, or de-briefing, and structured reflection opportunities, to enable you to process these feelings, which are after all understandable, and part of being human.

It is also important, if you feel you cannot give this man the care he needs, to inform a senior member, so that alternative persons can be involved if you feel out of your depth emotionally at this time. With the opportunity to reflect you may eventually feel that you are able to care for this man in a compassionate sense in the future. If we don't speak up when we feel uncomfortable then this can affect patients' experiences of care in a negative way. Patients may pick up on attitudes towards them either directly from non-verbal and verbal language or indirectly from avoidance tactics.

DAVID'S REFLECTIONS ON THIS SCENARIO

I agree with Vanessa's reasoning.

I would merely add a few comments about 'compassion' which is an extensively used word in healthcare. It's widely assumed that health professionals are and should be compassionate, but what 'compassion' is is not always clearly defined.

This is not the place for an in-depth philosophical analysis of compassion, though such an exercise would be helpful in a different context. However, I can open up a few points for reflection. It seems to me that:

- Compassion is a feeling, an emotion – something that is subjectively experienced.
- If we feel compassion then we must be able to imagine how things feel to another person, and have a sense of empathy and/or sympathy for him or her (though these words also need clarification).
- We may be mistaken in what we imagine, though as a health carer there are usually many opportunities to test out, for example via observation or simple questioning, whether what we imagine is close to the other person's experience.
- It's possible to pretend to be compassionate.
- There is an obvious difference between feeling compassion and acting on the feeling, for example actively helping another person out or feelings of empathy or sympathy. It might be argued that if we claim to feel compassion for others, for example needy children in the developing world, and yet do nothing to help them, then our feeling is either false or weak, whereas those people who both feel compassion and act on it are definitely compassionate.
- It's not easy – and may be impossible – to teach someone to be compassionate. I think it is definitely possible to help people understand better how other people are affected by life, and to encourage them to consider what it would be like to be the other person or to have their experiences (we commonly encourage children in this way), but if a person has no sense of the way life is for others, or simply doesn't care, then it is hard to see how this could be taught.
- It's sometimes argued that to be a health carer it is necessary to be compassionate, for example 'compassion' is one of the **6Cs** we reference in this book from time to time. But it seems to me that how you feel as a person towards the people for whom you are working for health is irrelevant, so long as you do a fair and balanced job. This is not to dismiss the importance of personal judgement, or our theory about it: we create **situations** as we interpret the world, as we explain in **Chapter Four**, but that does not mean that we should always react entirely subjectively and spontaneously to circumstances. If we subscribe to a developed theory of how one should act – in this case as a health worker – then we can and should apply this theory consistently. This would mean, for example, that if we do not like a patient then we ought to acknowledge this – we must be as self-aware as we can – but nonetheless apply the theory even-handedly.

I believe that some people in this world are able to feel compassion for anyone and everyone, while there are others who feel little or nothing for anyone other than themselves. However, both types can work for health if they choose, so long

(Continued)

as they adhere to a theory of health or rules of practice. That said, like most of us, I have been treated by health workers who felt no compassion towards me (or worse who were clearly disinterested in my plight) and by health workers who displayed and acted on genuine human concern. There is no doubt which sort I would rather be treated by – and not only that, but the effects on my confidence, feelings of being supported, and freedom to ask questions and for further help are always vastly more positive when I sense that my health carer feels real compassion toward me. (163)

SUGGESTION FOR SCENARIO 7.13: APPLY PSP TO THIS SCENARIO PLUS THE ETHICAL GRID AND INTUITION

—— SCENARIO 7.14: TIME TO TELL? ——

CATEGORIES: FORENSICS, LAW

Dean is a single man of 25. He is currently an inpatient, on remand, receiving care in the prison health service.

Dean has a diagnosis of antisocial personality disorder, and finds it incredibly difficult to trust anybody, in part due to considerable abuse and neglect as a young boy, which resulted in profound trauma and distress for him. Dean finds it difficult to manage his impulsive aggression towards others around him.

Before Dean's remand to prison, he killed a man who he suspected was planning to murder him. This is not in dispute.

Since admission, Dean has attempted to assault other staff and prisoners physically, and on one occasion, actually caused a serious injury to a staff member.

Following a detailed assessment, professionals at the local high secure unit have agreed to admit him. It is felt that this admission will more effectively meet his needs, and prevent any potential harm to others, before his trial.

The prison nurses wonder if they should tell Dean about the transfer immediately, or on the morning of his planned departure, in a week's time. He has previously stated 'If I'm transferred, I will smash up this place and everyone in it.'

People frequently say that one of their core values is honesty and truth – telling, so should Dean be told straight away? Or in a week's time, as he is about to be transferred? What if he asks you directly? What would you do?

EXAMPLE PROPOSAL FOR FOCUS: It is proposed that Dean is told immediately of his impending transfer to a high secure unit.

VANESSA'S REFLECTIONS ON THIS SCENARIO

While I don't agree that Dean should be told immediately, as I feel this needs to be a planned and well-thought out process, I agree he should be told as soon as possible, when safeguards and extra resources are in place.

Safety is a big consideration here, and there is a duty to protect the safety of others also – but just because Dean has made threats, it doesn't mean he will carry them out, although there is a real risk that he might.

There are many ways that Dean can be assisted in processing this information. Telling him at the earliest opportunity will assist in building trust and get him used to the idea, and allow time to explain why it is felt that the move will be beneficial for him.

If we wait for him to ask, then this would put professionals in a very difficult position. And if we wait for him to ask, and he is told at that point, there may not be the manpower or resources available to cope with any violence.

Dean may also become suspicious if he thinks details are being kept from him, or he is being lied to, and he may guess that something is about to change if staff start avoiding him or he is able to read non-verbal cues which are not congruent with what he is being told. I also think, in this circumstance, there is a risk that Dean will not receive the due care and attention that he deserves, morally, legally and professionally. This could also result in potential aggressive reactions.

Staff honesty is essential in establishing trust and building therapeutic relationships. If Dean is told as soon as possible then he is more likely to trust staff, both on his present ward and in his new service area. He may also take the opportunity to respond to open honesty, by revealing his own feelings and fears.

There is a further risk that if we are not honest in this situation, others in the unit will also wonder if staff are lying or keeping information from them, which could cause disharmony within the whole unit.

There is definitely an argument that lying is sometimes justified if is felt that the lie can avoid harm; however, I feel ultimately that both safety obligations and the individual rights of Dean can both be met with a well-thought out plan and extra contingencies put in place.

DAVID'S REFLECTIONS ON THIS SCENARIO

I agree entirely with Vanessa about this troubling issue.

According to my personal philosophy of health it is necessary, if you are to work for health, to serve needs first, respect people equally regardless of what they have

(Continued)

done or what you think of them, create their autonomy and respect their choices as far as this is possible and does not cause avoidable harm to others. In this case, this means to me, that while Dean does not appear to have a choice in where he will live, he does and should have other choices (for example, what food to eat or newspapers to read) and he should be empowered to have control over his life at every opportunity. Informing him clearly and as soon as is safely possible is therefore a requirement – this is a consequence of the philosophy I believe in and is also an immediate personal judgement: I would recoil from treating Dean differently from other people.

Note: This case study dilemma has been adapted from Coffey, M. and Byrt, R. (2010) *Forensic Mental Health Nursing, Ethics, Debates and Dilemmas*. London: Quay Books. (**136**)

SUGGESTION FOR SCENARIO 7.14: APPLY PSP TO THIS PLUS THE LAW AND VALUES-BASED DECISION-MAKING

SCENARIO 7.15: IT'S MY HOUSE AND I'LL SHARE IF I WANT TO

CATEGORIES: LAW, FAMILY

You are a community health professional. You are caring for an elderly male – Wesley – who's recently been diagnosed with mild dementia. Wesley has had life-long difficulties with social situations and relationships, demonstrating strong signs of Asperger's, which is a long-standing diagnosis.

Wesley has difficulty with complex activities of daily living but is able to perform all his personal care independently, when he wants to. A few years ago, a well-meaning ex-social worker – Gladys Jones – found Wesley living in squalor in a cockroach-infested house. She offered to move in and did a great job of cleaning the house – and has managed to maintain it over the years. Gladys has provided comprehensive care to Wesley, who is now physically in a much healthier state.

He is very stubborn and constantly plays pranks on Gladys and is certainly not easy to live with. It would be very difficult to find a carer with the patience to support him.

Last week, out of the blue, Gladys who provides three hours a week of funded support, has told you she is ready to resign and is considering leaving Wesley and the house.

Wesley's parents both passed away many years ago, leaving him a considerable inheritance including the four-bedroom house with two bathrooms on a large plot of land, where both he and Gladys currently reside.

Two years ago, Gladys convinced Wesley to sign over half the property to her. This came to the attention of the professional team at the time. They sought legal advice, which was that because Wesley was deemed to have the capacity to set up a will, he had every right to give away half his property. They did recommend that Wesley should appoint an independent Enduring Power of Attorney, who would act in Wesley's best interests, but he refused to do this.

You and your team have also been advised to apply to appoint a welfare guardian and have asked Wesley's social worker to assist with this. However, you do not have explicit consent for this move either.

It is obvious that Wesley cares a great deal for Gladys, but it does not seem to be an equal relationship. You feel that Gladys is manipulating Wesley by threatening to leave. She is explicitly keen for you to continue to provide therapy to enable greater independence, and she does seem to be supporting his best interests. Yet you feel uneasy about her intentions.

You've noticed that Wesley frequently changes his answers to your questions when Gladys is not present. He also confides that he finds her moods difficult to manage. Nonetheless, he will do anything to keep her in the house – he couldn't possibly cope without her and would be desolate if she left, he says. Over the years, various attempts to teach him to be more assertive have not worked.

Your assessment is that Wesley is not able to live independently. You consider that he would be better living in care. He already enjoys attending a day programme at a rest home three times a week, but Wesley is adamant that he will not leave his family home. Due to his Asperger's he finds it extremely difficult to adjust to change. And it is undoubtedly the case that he would be devastated to be separated from his friend.

What would you do in this situation? Would a welfare guardian be able to protect Wesley's best interests, if Gladys remains in the house full time?

Should Wesley be allowed to live where he wants, despite evidence of manipulative behaviour from Gladys?

Should you recommend that Wesley moves to residential care?

Do you agree with the proposal below?

EXAMPLE PROPOSAL FOR FOCUS: It is proposed that the client is supported to live in the family home with his friend but be appointed a welfare guardian even if he doesn't want one.

VANESSA'S REFLECTIONS ON THIS SCENARIO

After some slow thinking I find that I disagree with the proposal, although I do have some concerns about Wesley's situation and his relationship with Gladys. Overall,

(Continued)

however, it is not my business to override his wishes if he is capable of understanding and making his own choices. A welfare guardian can be applied for in a court by anyone with an interest in Wesley, but only if he lacks capacity. At present, there is no evidence that he does.

Wesley has made his intentions and wishes clear. He would like to remain living at home and has no doubts about that at all. He is also refusing to be assigned a Power of Attorney, as is his right.

In this scenario, I would take an enabling approach in the first instance. Although Wesley has capacity there is a certain amount of vulnerability associated with Asperger's and his recent dementia diagnosis, so he may need assistance to enhance his ability to make an independent decision, and perhaps to assert himself with certain individuals, if he feels he might be being manipulated.

After careful discussion Wesley might agree to try a welfare guardian, with a review of the situation at three-monthly intervals so that he knows he can change his mind if he has the capacity to do so. Having said that, I think his existing social worker is most appropriate at present.

I would also talk to Wesley about ensuring that he makes his boundaries clear with Gladys, regarding what is acceptable to him and what isn't. And that if anything concerns him about her behaviour or actions then he is free to speak to a professional at any time to assist in empowering him to assert his wishes and have his needs met by others.

DAVID'S REFLECTIONS ON THIS SCENARIO

Fast thinking is probably too fast in this apparently complex case, but for me, despite the detail, I think this issue is reasonably straightforward. The key factors that spring out to me are:

- Wesley wants to stay in the house
- Gladys has cared well for Wesley but is thinking of resigning and leaving
- Wesley does not want her to leave
- Wesley needs support
- 'You' think he would be better in full-time care
- 'You' think Gladys is manipulating Wesley

It seems to me that not all of these factors are relevant to you as a health worker. Though you may feel they are, this emphasis is clearly from you as a **person** and other persons may well see the circumstances very differently.

Whether or not Gladys has manipulated Wesley – and vice versa – seems impossible to establish. They have a long-standing relationship and in any such bonding who has manipulated who, in what ways and why and for how long, are open questions, beyond your scope.

Given this, we are left with a situation where Wesley's carer may leave, we know he needs support, so it seems only sensible to appoint a welfare guardian, but only if Wesley wants one, and finds rapport with the potential guardian. If he or she is competent and professional then he will be able to offer support to Wesley, including helping him process Gladys' impending or actual departure, and overall creating and respecting his autonomy to help him live the best life he can as things move on.

I do wonder why the social worker is not offering more help and support, and I would want to understand this better if I could.

Overall, I agree with the proposal since Wesley does seem vulnerable – or potentially vulnerable – but Wesley must agree and there is work to be done to support him to consider this option. I would want to share this work with the social worker if possible.

SUGGESTION FOR SCENARIO 7.15: APPLY PSP TO THIS SCENARIO PLUS THE LAW AND RISK ANALYSIS

SCENARIO 7.16: RICHARD — THE TEENAGER WITH A SECRET ...

CATEGORIES: LAW, CONFIDENTIALITY

Richard, recently turned 15, is a student at a mainstream Catholic High School.

Richard's mother, Alison, has become concerned that Richard has not been 'acting like himself'. She has noticed that he has become increasingly withdrawn, secretive and uncommunicative over the past few months. She realises that this is not unusual for a mid-teenager, but her mother's 'intuition' is causing alarm bells to ring.

Alison has arranged for Richard to see his pediatrician, Dr Karen Moore, who Richard knows well, for a follow-up appointment for an unrelated issue, concerning previous chronic ear infections that now seem to be under control.

Before Dr Moore steps in to see Richard alone, Alison pulls her to one side. She expresses briefly her worries, telling the doctor, 'I know he trusts you. If you can please find out what's troubling him please tell me. I really feel he needs our help.'

(Continued)

After some coaxing and gentle questioning, Richard reveals that he has become romantically and sexually involved with another boy at school. Then he blurts out, 'I'm really scared I've caught something from him, it's messing up my life.' When Dr Moore starts to talk about his mother, and her concerns about his low mood, Richard immediately looks very anxious. He implores the doctor not to reveal what he has told her, but just to help him. He says, 'Please don't tell her, she doesn't have to know. She's really against homosexuality – she calls us "queers" and worse, whenever the subject crops up in the media or conversation. It's a terrible situation, please just help me.'

What do you think should be done? Do you agree with the proposal below?

EXAMPLE PROPOSAL FOR FOCUS: It is proposed that Dr Moore informs Richard's mother of what Richard has disclosed.

VANESSA'S REFLECTIONS ON THIS SCENARIO

My fast thinking reaction to this scenario is that I don't think the doctor would be justified in disclosing any information to Richard's mother at present. There are professional, legal and ethical issues to consider, which I try to clarify below, while also trying to imagine the different **situations** created by those most closely involved.

RICHARD'S SITUATION

Richard is very anxious that his mother will find out his secret especially as, according to him, she has made homophobic remarks in the past.

We can assume that Richard will be worried that his mum may reject him because of his sexual orientation, and therefore not show unconditional love and acceptance, which is very important for any child. Richard is also worried that he has caught a sexually transmitted disease (STD) from his romantic partner, which must be causing him great anxiety. Richard will probably be feeling embarrassed, scared and possibly ashamed, even disclosing to the doctor he trusts, given that he belongs to a family who have normalised frequent homophobic comments as acceptable.

Richard has a legal right to confidentiality from the doctor treating him. There are exceptions; however, a breach of this obligation from professionals can only reasonably be defended under certain circumstances.

Despite only being 15, he also has a legal right to a private life according to the Human Rights Act 1998, Article 8, which further emphasises the importance of keeping sensitive information private, even from his mother.

MOTHER'S SITUATION

Imagining the picture from Mum's point of view is hard, as we don't know much about her apart from what Richard has said. I feel cross with her for making comments to Richard about homosexuality, because now he feels he can't speak about his health concerns. However, as a mother of two teenage boys myself, I can imagine how concerned she would feel if she knew intuitively something was wrong and her son didn't feel able to divulge or share with her.

Although it is normal for teenagers to withhold some information from their parents, Richard's mother may feel like he doesn't trust her or that it might be a serious issue or secret if he is not prepared to share it with her. She has built up a relationship of trust with the doctor and expects her to share with her if it's something important she should be aware of.

THE DOCTOR'S SITUATION

I imagine that having built up a relationship with Richard and his mother over the years the doctor would naturally feel concern for both. However, her duty is first and foremost to Richard in this instance. She is obliged to keep Richard's confidence, and only disclose under certain specified conditions.

Confidence can be breached under the following circumstances:

- With Richard's explicit consent
- If this involves sharing information with others involved in care and treatment, which is necessary for the performance of their duties, with consent
- Disclosure in the interests of justice
- Disclosure in the public interest to do so
- Disclosure to protect a third party – this does not apply to Richard's mother in this instance but might apply to a sexual partner if an STD were diagnosed
- Disclosure to prevent or detect a serious crime. (164)

WHAT WOULD I DO IF I WERE THE DOCTOR?

I would reassure Richard that no disclosure would be made, but I would also encourage him to try to find a way to share information with his mother if possible, as it would release a lot of anxiety for him. Having said that, it is also ok for him to choose not to, and I would tell him that.

I think a way forward would be to gain his consent to refer on to a therapist or a professional who could assist him in how to tackle his anxieties about this subject, and this might give him the confidence to eventually disclose his secret to his family, or at least be able to challenge their beliefs and comments in a way which educates and fosters tolerance for diversity.

If Mum asks the doctor what has been said, she can empathise but clearly explain that she is obliged to keep his confidence. She can explain that if Richard wishes to

(Continued)

disclose anything then this is his choice. If Mum asks Richard what the doctor said then he could simply refuse to say or he could tell her, and ask her to respect his privacy for example, or say that he is being referred for 'talk therapy' for anxiety – or whatever he wishes to say, since this is his choice and responsibility.

Were Richard to require treatment then the scenario would be different. Normally, a parent would be expected to consent on behalf of the minor. However, given the confidentiality issue, it is likely that the health professionals would apply 'Gillick competence'. (**165**)

DAVID'S REFLECTIONS ON THIS SCENARIO

In this case the suggested approach below makes good sense.

With regard to the law, what to do is left to your personal judgement, though there are rules that you need to consider. The legal situation, according to the General Medical Council (**GMC**), is basically that you should protect confidential information in the same way you would for an adult, i.e. you should assume capacity, however there are circumstances in which you can disclose:

SHARING INFORMATION WITHOUT CONSENT

If a child or young person does not agree to disclosure there are still circumstances in which you should disclose information:

a.   when there is an overriding public interest in the disclosure
b.   when you judge that the disclosure is in the best interests of a child or young person who does not have the maturity or understanding to make a decision about disclosure
c.   when disclosure is required by law. (**166**)

These provisos, of course, also require personal judgement to be interpreted, but the general tone seems to be that if the young person is able to understand his situation in the way an adult would, you ought to respect his wishes.

How you see this set of circumstances will vary according to your values, what you are as a person, your view of childhood or youth – there are all sorts of factors it's important to be aware of. It will also depend on how you see your role as a health professional, and who you think the primary patient is – the mother or the son? If you see the situation as Alison does – perhaps you have children of a similar age, and perhaps you too are naturally protective – then you may want to talk to her about Richard's circumstances. If you see the situation as being little or nothing to do with the mother then you will work with Richard alone, to support and assist him, as an independent individual.

If I were the doctor in this case then **PSP** would be helpful, particularly to help me identify my own values and prejudices, and I would use it with Richard to identify as much as possible how he sees himself as a **person** and his **situation**. I would then work with that and try to establish clinical and legal facts with and for Richard, try to explore his anxieties and look at what he would like to happen ideally. I would consider myself Richard's baseline health worker but I would bring in other professionals and resources as needed.

So, I would ask questions and, if indicated, physically investigate whether he has 'caught something', and move on from there according to what I found. I would also recommend counselling to Richard, on his own at first.

I would ask Richard directly if he would like to involve his mother and if not I would respect that. I would tell her that Richard has asked me to help him as a professional and does not want anything passed on from this process, as is his right. I would give her information to read about Richard's rights.

I would not tell Alison what Richard has disclosed to me but I would make my very best efforts to create autonomy for Richard and to work out ways, with him, of achieving a much happier and more positive set of circumstances.

SUGGESTION FOR SCENARIO 7.16: APPLY PSP TO THIS SCENARIO PLUS VALUES-BASED DECISION-MAKING AND/OR THE LAW

—— SCENARIO 7.17: LEAVE ME ALONE! ——

CATEGORIES: CAPACITY, CONSENT, TERMINAL ILLNESS

Audrey is a frail 98-year-old who's been living in a care home since the death of her husband, Bob, 12 months ago. Audrey and Bob were married for 70 years. Audrey now has no surviving family or friends and values her privacy and independence, rarely choosing to join in with communal day-room activities.

Audrey's always preferred to eat her meals in her room, but lately she's been eating less and less. In the last week, Audrey's stopped eating all together. She says she's had enough of life. She feels sad and lonely. The only thing she wants is to 'join her husband in heaven'. It has been suggested to her that she could be fed in other ways, which she found shocking and immediately refused to consider.

(Continued)

It's assumed that Audrey has capacity (in law). She does not have a terminal illness, but she suffers with long-standing and severe arthritis, which limits her mobility. Her condition has deteriorated significantly over the last 12 months. Audrey has lost 6 kg in the last two weeks. She currently weighs 55 kg, and is drinking water only.

You're the health professional in charge of Audrey's care. You have a dilemma: if you respect Audrey's wishes then you will be contributing to her demise, if you force her to take nutrition via alternative means, such as a parenteral feed, then you will be sustaining her life but going against her clearly stated preference.

What would you do in this situation?

EXAMPLE PROPOSAL FOR FOCUS: It is proposed that you respect Audrey's wishes.

VANESSA'S REFLECTIONS ON THIS SCENARIO

I feel that there isn't enough information for me to decide conclusively what to do at present. I would want to know if this is a temporary setback due to a reactive depression, and what has been tried to tempt her to regain interest in socialising and in nutrition.

Maybe carers could find a way of keeping her company in her room, maybe playing a card game or similar, or looking at photographs of her husband with her, to enable her to process her talk about him and process her grief.

I would most likely encourage Audrey to try and eat refreshing foods. It needn't be much, even small things such as grapes may make her mouth feel fresher and food more palatable to her – this might improve her appetite. There are also other questions that need to be asked: Is she not eating because her mouth is sore? Is she constipated? Has she had bereavement support? Has she been offered medication? Her lack of motivation and interest could have various causes, and I wouldn't want to withhold attempts at getting her to take food on the information given. If on presentation of a variety of foods, Audrey still refused to eat, then that is her choice to make, but I'd hope the option would continue to be offered.

Ultimately, if all has failed and Audrey has been given treatment options and choices and she still declines then I would follow her wishes and try to make her as comfortable as possible. It's assumed in law that she has capacity at present, and so to force her to eat would be contrary to this, and would also be a breach of her human rights, no matter how benevolent the intent.

Audrey has lived a long life. I've seen widows and widowers who are left behind give up many times, and I truly believe that in their hearts that life holds no further interest for them and they just want to be with their loved ones who have passed.

DAVID'S REFLECTIONS ON THIS SCENARIO

I agree with Vanessa about this scenario.

Using **PSP** – just like using other ways of attempting empathy – brings with it the danger of projecting one's own self and views on other people. I am not yet 98, can't imagine being 98 (don't want to be 98), but can well imagine, that were I to have no autonomy, no prospects and constant feelings of deep sadness I would not want to carry on.

This is what Audrey has asked for essentially. Legally I cannot force her to eat and ethically, the way I see it using the Grid, while I would want to persist with efforts to create autonomy for Audrey – as Vanessa describes – I would also want to respect her autonomy – her choice not to eat any more.

I would support her and make her as comfortable as I could and I would talk to her about Bob and the past if I could and she wanted to talk. I would respect Audrey's wishes.

SUGGESTION FOR SCENARIO 7.17: APPLY PSP TO THIS SCENARIO PLUS THE LAW AND ETHICAL GRID

SCENARIO 7.18: DEALING WITH RACIST VIEWS

CATEGORIES: VALUES, PROFESSIONAL ROLE, RACISM

When someone you're counselling divulges what many people would consider offensive racial views, should you continue to see the client?

Tim is a 45-year-old man who's sought counselling from you for low self-esteem and depression. During the first few sessions Tim was quietly spoken. It was initially difficult for you to build rapport.

However, you've been seeing Tim for several weeks now and have established what you perceive to be a solid and safe working relationship. Tim now seems to trust you sufficiently to be able to open up and discuss deep problems he's been harbouring for many years.

(Continued)

As a therapist, you regularly find yourself working with clients with different values from your own, but always aim to make the client feel accepted in order to foster the therapeutic relationship.

The problem is that now he's more at ease with you, Tim's demonstrating extreme negative feelings towards some cultural groups. He feels increasingly free to make racist comments, some of which you find extreme.

You want to continue to help Tim, and have agreed future sessions, but at the same time you're finding it difficult to know what to do about his adverse feelings towards others.

While you see the importance of accepting the client's views, you wonder if it compromises your responsibility to those outside the client –counsellor relationship.

Do you agree with the proposal below?

EXAMPLE PROPOSAL FOR FOCUS: It is proposed that you ignore Tim's racist comments and continue with therapy as usual.

VANESSA'S REFLECTIONS ON THIS SCENARIO

I think the therapist has a professional responsibility not to judge individual patients (easier said than done) but rather to help them approach their problems in a more positive way. The fact that Tim is exhibiting 'racist behaviour' in expressing his views should not affect the way the therapist deals with him, as he deserves just as much respect as anyone else. The therapist has a duty, I believe, to acknowledge her personal feelings, whatever they are, but to try to put these aside as far as delivering clinical care is concerned. This doesn't mean that you have to condone a view you disagree with but, in my opinion, the most important ideal at present is trust. Tim trusts the therapist not to judge him and his views but rather help him. He also trusts that his personal views should not affect the way he is treated.

The goal of improving Tim's mental health is uppermost for me and to openly show repulsion for his views could be counterproductive to his recovery at this stage. Having said that, I do not believe that these extreme views should be ignored entirely. I would continue to work with Tim as the relationship progresses and guide him to explore where these views came from, prompting him to think about the people he knows and to look more deeply at what is driving him, as a person.

If Tim were incapable of reviewing his thought process and not ready to be openly challenged, I would consider setting him some homework, such as reading articles on Black History and examples of positive contributions those of other races have made to Western culture, industry and peoples. Gently challenging him, when he is ready, is the way forward in my view. This may help him become more tolerant of others, deal with his anger towards those of a different race and culture, and see things from others' perspectives.

DAVID'S REFLECTIONS ON THIS SCENARIO

This is a complex and difficult matter. Tim has asked me to counsel him and I wish to help him, and he has recently started to express very negative views towards cultures other than his own. I do not share his views.

I was tempted to say that I don't see Tim's racism as a health work issue – that it is beyond the scope of health work. But I feel that this would be an arbitrary choice. I think, especially where mental health is concerned, I should consider every factor that makes Tim the **person** he is at the moment, and at the same time I need to be as aware as possible of myself as a **person**, not least so that I do not discriminate negatively against Tim because of his views.

Given that this is a counselling scenario I would encourage Tim to examine all his views, prejudices and life experiences and I would focus on those that seem of most significance to his circumstances and his future well-being. I would tell him where I disagree with him, but say that I am not judging him at all, just trying to help him explore how he has arrived where he is. I would ask open questions designed to help him reflect on all his views and all his life, including his racism.

SUGGESTION FOR SCENARIO 7.18: APPLY PSP PLUS TO THIS SCENARIO PLUS THE ETHICAL GRID

SUMMARY OF CHAPTERS SIX AND SEVEN

These practical chapters have offered a range of real-life scenarios on which to practise **PSP PLUS**, or any other form of personal judgement you favour. These scenarios provide invaluable practice in careful reflection in conditions of uncertainty, where there are no right answers to be had.

The scenarios support and evidence our theoretical discussion in other chapters.

CHAPTERS SIX AND SEVEN EXERCISES

Having read **Chapters Six and Seven** you may like to attempt the following exercises, to reinforce your learning:

1. Register on the Values Exchange provided for a companion book in this series: https://thoughtful. vxcommunity.com/
2. Respond online to at least one scenario and review the results
3. Take a scenario from the present chapter (above) and analyse it using the strategy suggested
4. If you are working with other students consider their opinions about and justifications of at least one scenario in this chapter – notice how they create different **situations** from you
5. In how many scenarios did you change your mind from your initial or 'gut' reaction? If you changed your mind, why did you do this?

CHAPTER 8

USING IMAGINATION TO IMPROVE PERSONAL JUDGEMENT

AIMS

This chapter has the following aims:

1) To present various ways to try to see the world as others see it
2) To offer the **Rings of Uncertainty** as one method that you and others may find helpful
3) To show how just a few changes in persons and/or circumstances can make a massive difference to our perceptions, using the case of Tilly from **Chapter Four**
4) To further explain and justify the belief that there is no 'bird's eye view' in nursing and healthcare decision-making
5) To argue that since personal judgement is a partly mysterious process that happens constantly and everywhere, reflection about it and practice with it should be a substantial component of all health and nursing education

LEARNING OUTCOMES

When you have worked through this chapter you should be able to:

1) Better appreciate the importance of trying to see the world through other people's eyes
2) Understand the Rings of Uncertainty
3) Apply the **Rings of Uncertainty** to any healthcare circumstances
4) Understand the full implications of the **Train Journey** we describe in **Chapter Three**

CHOOSE A WAY OF JUDGING THAT WORKS FOR YOU

We have seen that while there are various ways to make decisions in nursing and healthcare, they each have significant limitations and none can be applied without a personal decision to do so. There are algorithms, rules and processes – each of the nursing models we outline in **Chapter One** has these – but there is always a need for personal judgement, to choose the model, interpret it in context, and apply it in practice. Often in everyday circumstances there is no obvious method, in which case everything is left to personal judgement; fast, slow or any other speed.

Because personal judgements are inescapable in nursing and healthcare, and because there's no ideal method of making them, it's worth trying any approach that might work for you:

Although there is no universal formula for making better decisions, good judgment is key ... it is 'the faculty of mind by which order is perceived in a situation previously considered disordered.' Basically, good judgment ... (enables) ... you to find patterns and predict meaningful events. (**167**)

What you have to do, we think, is not only find order in the world, but try to work out **why** you find that particular order (what is it about you that sees this way? What is it about you that sees this pattern or this meaning?) And, we believe, you must also try – as much as you possibly can – to work out what orders, patterns and meanings other people see.

EXAMPLES

We're not alone in what we suggest – there are many others who understand the limits of objectified, 'target-based healthcare' and who try to work out how better to understand the intricacies of entwined patient and carer realities. These approaches take effort to apply since everyone and every situation is different – but they are infinitely more creative, imaginative and caring than flow charts and check boxes – which may seem technical, rigorous and consistent, but which in truth are trivial distortions of real life.

Bill Fulford's values-based practice, for example, is designed to enable those involved in caring – both staff and clients – to see what matters most to each other, and to work out together what to do for the best when they find that their values clash (**113**).

The **Point of Care Foundation** has three programmes, each of which in various ways is designed to help everyone better understand the worlds of others (**168**). One approach is particularly interesting. It's called the Sweeney Programme, which grew out of Dr Kieran Sweeney's own experience as a cancer patient (**169**). In his moving personal account, the late doctor says:

> ... medicine is not solely a technical activity and pursuit, medicine is about understanding and being with people at the edge of the human predicament ... it's the relational care where the experience has been less than satisfactory ...

The Sweeney Programme believes that staff can provide the best care by stepping back and seeing experiences through the patient's eyes, and offers education and tools to equip staff to do this. The programme assists staff to step into patients' shoes, using tested and effective tools, in order to help them get as close to experiencing the patient's journey as possible (**170**).

Expounding a similar ethos to our own:

> The programme is born out of the belief that relational aspects of care are as important as the technical clinical aspects, but that these aspects often get neglected. While healthcare staff are motivated to care, it takes conscious and sustained effort to understand the patient's experience and consider their fears, vulnerabilities and needs as an individual. Staff can only consider what matters most to the patient, and then change their actions accordingly, if they are given the space, time, and resources to understand the patient's perspective. (**171**)

A participant in the programme, Joanne Minford, eloquently describes the benefits for her:

> The methods used in the Sweeney programme really did change the way I thought about what was important to patients navigating through NHS care and how much what we experience might affect compliance with, and the success of, our treatment. For me the relentless drive to be efficient in target-based healthcare culture totally missed the point of caring and the programme was my antidote. Now, having had my own 'care experience', I really appreciate the power of these methods in refocusing us around the personal, around not only the effects of the treatment we deliver but of how we deliver that treatment, and around what is truly of value to our patients and their families. (**172**)

Further very useful resources – all of which are designed to support and foster personal judgement – may be discovered here (**173**).

When she was a practising nurse, Vanessa would try to include personal elements by drawing or imagining an image with 'the patient' at the centre and various considerations surrounding him or her. These considerations could be anything relevant, but were most often concepts like 'risk', 'law' and 'ethics' that Vanessa could reflect on personally, and which she could also share and discuss with the patient and her colleagues, as required.

In addition, there are multiple general advice books and online sites about how to make decisions, most of which have common threads with our own thinking in this book. For example, wikiHow talks about 'framing decisions', being aware of your emotions, weighing pros and cons, and looking at a choice from different perspectives (**174**). However, it also suggests 'removing yourself from the decision' and trying not to be personally 'involved', which we think is striving in vain for an unattainable objective vantage point.

How we Decide by Jonah Lehrer gives interesting examples and an informative discussion about the uncertainties and unknowables of decision-making (**25**), concluding, as we do, that practice and conversation with others rather than endless analysis is the best way to make better decisions, assuming that it really is possible to establish what 'better decisions' are:

> The simple truth of the matter is that making good decisions requires us to use both sides of the mind. For too long, we've treated human nature as an either/or situation. We are either rational or irrational. We either rely on statistics or trust our gut instincts. There's Apollonian logic versus Dionysian feeling; the id against the ego; the reptilian brain fighting the frontal lobes.
>
> Not only are these dichotomies false, they're destructive. There is no universal solution to the problem of decision-making. The real world is just too complex. As a result, natural selection endowed us with a brain that is enthusiastically pluralistic. Sometimes we need to reason through options and carefully analyse the possibilities. And sometimes we need to listen to our emotions. The secret is knowing when to use these different styles of thought. We always need to be thinking how we think.

Lehrer recommends taking a process from the aviation industry – called Cockpit Resource Management (**CRM**) and extending it into more and more areas of decision-making. **CRM** is essentially a way to create an environment where a diversity of viewpoints is freely shared.

This approach is obviously sensible, but has many limitations, not least that it's most useful where collective wisdom can lead to testable, 'right answers', such as those required in the airline industry and in clinical decision-making in healthcare. It's much less obviously useful for the type of real-life decision-making we have discussed in this book. But it's definitely a technique that could be used within groups that have the time and desire to work together to improve personal judgement.

THE RINGS OF UNCERTAINTY

As a final support, we offer one further way to use imagination to picture situations in a way that might be conveyed to others, and that others might convey to you: the **Rings of Uncertainty** – a device one of us came up with some years ago (**175**).

The Rings are an attempt to help people picture how they and others understand **situations**.

Though far from perfect, the idea is simple enough. A person using the Rings should first identify a problem (or **situation**, to use the present book's terminology) and then picture him or herself standing in a set of Rings, as if on a large plastic mat, perhaps:

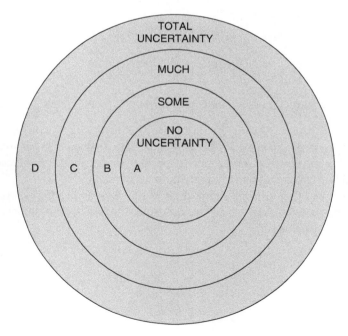

Figure 8.1   The Rings of Uncertainty

The Rings suggest an initial focus: how certain am I about this situation? How certain am I that I can intervene well? How confident am I that I can create a good outcome?

For example, do I have specialist competence in this situation (A)? Do I need support from colleagues or others (B)? Is collaboration essential (C)? Or am I incompetent to deal with this (D)?

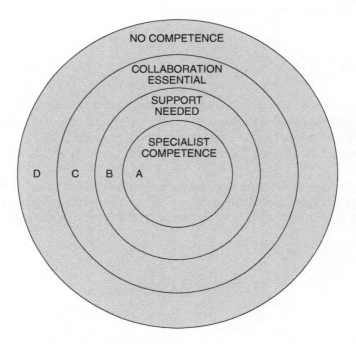

Figure 8.2   The Rings Expressed for Competence

The person reflecting should place herself – either with a marker or in her imagination – in whichever Ring she feel best represents her position in the situation. She can also invite others, including colleagues and the patient, to do the same.

All involved can then further define their positions by indicating where they stand within the Rings in relation to further key concepts. The five options below were offered in the original book chapter:

- Competence
- Resources
- Law
- Communication
- Ethics

For example:

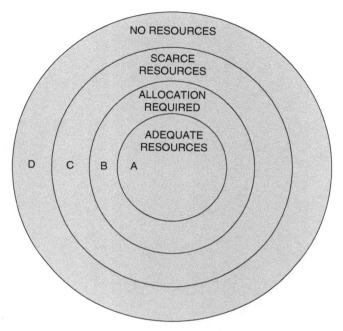

Figure 8.3   The Rings Expressed for Resources

And for law:

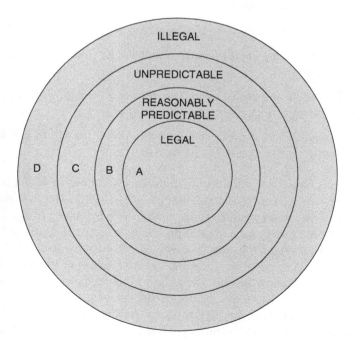

Figure 8.4   The Rings Expressed for Law

For communication:

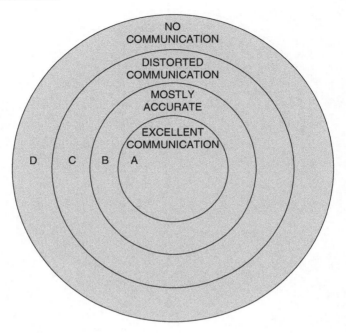

Figure 8.5   The Rings Expressed for Communication

And for ethics the levels were (moving from the outer Ring inwards):

D: Immoral policy (for example, prescribing inappropriate medication for a disliked patient)

C: Morally dubious policy – area of much controversy (for example, selling one of your kidneys, euthanasia)

B: Generally morally acceptable policy (for example, funding healthcare to all who need it free of charge funded by compulsory taxation)

A: Uncontroversially moral policy (for example, saving the life of a stranger in an emergency when no one else will be harmed as a result)

Of course, this idea is almost arbitrary. Different definitions of each concept could be used, and alternative concepts altogether could be featured. But this is not really a problem – if other ways are preferred and found to help in judging situations then this is good. In the end it's up to each of us to decide in our own ways, after all.

What really matters about the Rings, and why we've chosen to reincarnate this thinking tool, is that there has to be imagination and picturing to use it: the Rings are not just words, not just ideas, not just analysis. Rather, using them requires **you**, a unique person, to place yourself in the image – to imagine yourself stepping into the Rings, rather like a health professional Alice stepping gingerly onto a Looking Glass chess board.

To develop the picturing process further, anyone using the Rings can put the concepts together, as wedges, like this:

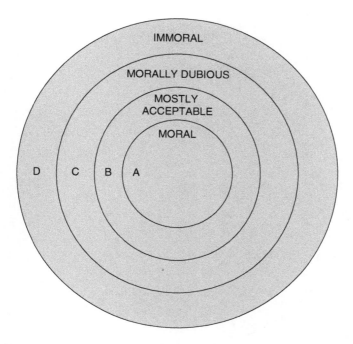

Figure 8.6   The Rings Expressed for Ethics

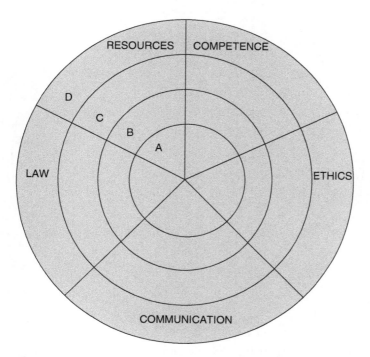

Figure 8.7   The Rings Fully Expressed

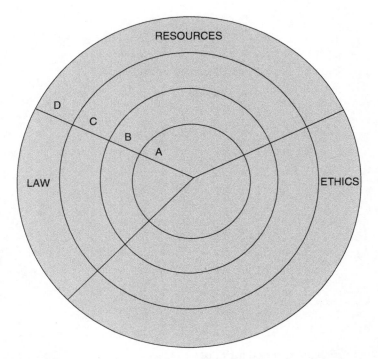

Figure 8.8   The Rings in Use to Reflect on Where one Stands

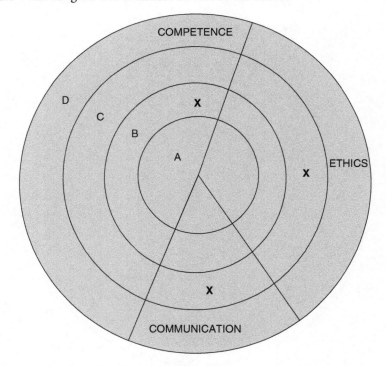

Figure 8.9   Wassim's Rings at This Point in Time

The person judging can choose to use a wedge or not, and can change the relative size of each to reflect her view of their importance to the situation (see **Figure 8.7**).

The person may place dots or crosses in each section, to represent her personal impression of where she stands (see **Figure 8.8**).

In Joe's case (see **Chapters Two** and **Four**) for example, Wassim – who's written a thesis on the ethics of dementia – might create a view like this to reflect where he stands and, therefore, convey at least part of the basis of his personal judgement (see **Figure 8.9**).

Wassim does not feel fully competent in this situation, and by choosing **B** is indicating a need for support from colleagues. And by setting this wedge at about 50% Wassim is also indicating that this is the most important aspect of the situation for him, at this moment. He's also aware that whatever he decides will be ethically controversial (**C**) and that his communication with Joe is likely to be distorted at best (**C**).

Fatima, on the other hand, has known Joe for 20 years. She does not see him only as an old man with dementia. She recognises Joe the person and is immediately clear that she should tell him the truth. Accordingly, Fatima may imagine a personal picture like the one shown in **Figure 8.10**.

Fatima's picture of her judgement is very different from Wassim's. She decides intuitively to tell him his wife is dead, and she supports this, both instinctively and on reflection, with the beliefs that to do so is legal (which it is), that her decision will be morally acceptable to most people (which is arguable), and that as a specialist in dementia care she is fully competent in this situation. She also believes she can communicate adequately with Joe.

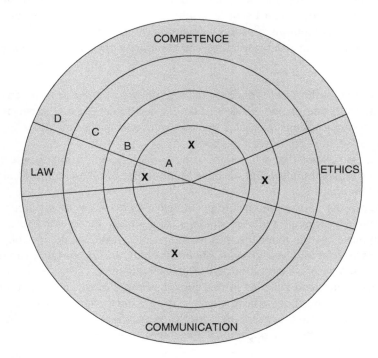

Figure 8.10   Fatima's Rings at This Point in Time

Used this way the Rings are a simple way to clarify further what you as a person bring to the situation. They can be used to excellent effect in teamwork. Each person can share her imaginative view of herself with others in the team. The different views can even be superimposed, to highlight areas of agreement and difference.

But whatever device you use, you must be aware that the **TRUTH** will be forever elusive. Personal judgement is not a process one can accurately specify. Rather, it is a dynamic process of acting, thinking and feeling, justifying and revising. It's a process of perpetual change – not linear, not prescribable, and not particularly teachable. Personal judgement is a personal experience and a personal task: if you want to make better personal judgements then you need to observe yourself as you make your decisions, and as you practise with our 43 scenarios, if this is what you choose to do.

In the end, only you are in charge of your personal judgement.

THERE IS NO BIRD'S EYE VIEW

Early in this book we briefly discuss a 'mythical decision-maker':

> This fictional creature is able to detach herself from what's going on around her, even emotionally. Her values and drives are permanent and predictable, and barely affected by her circumstances. She is willing and able to apply the best standards – clinically and ethically – to arrive at the right answers, of which in most cases there can be little doubt. Whatever happens, she will 'keep her head'. This fabulous person can even be ethical in an impersonal way, by behaving in line with ethical codes and standard policies, just as every other 'ethical person' can.

We are aware that this view of decision-making remains popular. In common law and in the professions the autonomous, fully responsible decision-maker is regarded as supreme: an ultimately detached individual able to calmly work out what is best, according to official standards – the 'buck stops' with this person.

We are also aware that a book about personal judgement might be expected to somehow support this view. But we have found things to be much more complex and entangled than this.

We do see the person who has to decide what to do in any given circumstance as central. We're individuals and at most stages of life when faced with choices we have no option other than to make these as individuals. However, we do not and cannot do this unconnected from a vast array of influences on us, and we certainly can never take a bird's eye view, as if we are untouched by these influences.

We have found, and included in this book, a number of complexities that begin to reveal the true reality of personal judgement. We believe it's vital for the best healthcare education and practice that these are understood as fully as possible, so that we can all properly appreciate the role of personal judgement, as it really is.

In sum, these are:

1. People are incredibly complex, varied and changeable. We are influenced by many different factors, in constantly changing proportion, and we are mostly unaware of these factors, how their balance changes, and how they affect us. When we don't think about it we're inclined to see ourselves as the 'mythical decision-maker'. But this is a delusion, as shown by **Figure 8.11**, presented earlier and repeated here:

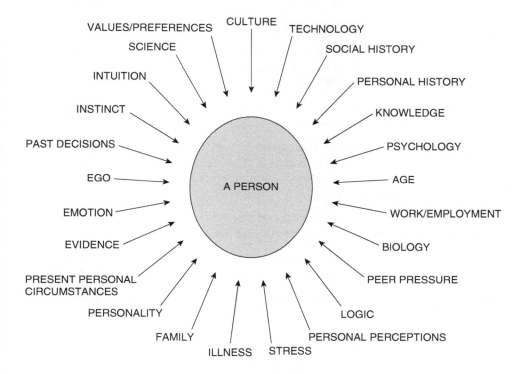

Figure 8.11   Some Influences that Create Persons

2. Our circumstances are at least as complex as we are. In order to cope with such complexity we simplify what we experience, and focus on those aspects of the circumstances that we can most easily comprehend and affect. This tendency is well known as 'bias' in psychology, and includes 'confirmation bias' in which we look for evidence to confirm our beliefs and discount other evidence, and 'group think' where only the ideas seen to be valid by the members of the group are allowed and the harmony of the group is more important than the individual perspective **(123)**.
3. When judgement is needed in life, we combine highly complex selves with highly complex circumstances to create a unique view of reality, which we call **situations** in this book. Because of the 'bird's eye view' fallacy we tend to believe that others see the same situation as we do, but this is never true.
4. There is a massive 'grey area' of decision-making both in nursing and life in general where it's simply unclear what it is best to do and where we must make choices. We argue we must make these choices accepting the reality of how and why we judge – only then can we make true improvements in our ability to judge well.

5. We find that the slightest changes in ourselves and/or our circumstances can bring about massive changes in perceived situations. For example, in **Scenario 4.1** in **Chapter Four** we describe university students' reactions to a 'family in crisis'. We asked them who is the most important family member to focus on, as a health carer. A young man called Rob was clearly selected.

    A second cohort of different students, a few months later, was asked almost the same question, but with a few changes:

    > Dad, Stuart is not coping as a newly single parent bringing up his teenage son, Rob and pregnant teenage daughter, Tilly. He is not looking after himself properly and appears to be drinking.

    > Son, Rob is not coping well with his mum's death and has stopped opening up to anyone. He has just had a head injury after falling off his bike.

    > Daughter, Teenager Tilly is pregnant and appears to have mild learning difficulties. She is struggling to cope with being pregnant or understand what is happening to her. The father was met online and is no longer around. She has a pain in her stomach.

    > Grannie Betty cares for her husband Bert. She has just fallen down the stairs and appears to have sustained injuries to her ankle, hip and head.

    > Grandpa Bert has Alzheimer's and does not say much at all. Cannot attend to personal care without help and encouragement. (**Credit Tim Howell, the University of Derby**)

    When asked who is most important, there was a completely different result:

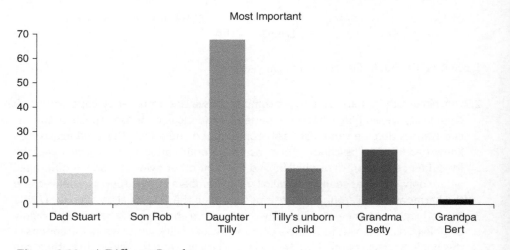

Figure 8.12   A Different Result

Son Rob, previously far and away of most concern, is now of second least concern, way behind Tilly, and yet he still has the same head injury that was so troubling to the first cohort.

Some of the circumstances have changed, and this has made an enormous difference to the personal judgements of the students.

Both cohorts were able to view the results as they came in, and it is therefore possible that they followed and firmed up early trends, in a form of group think. But, if so, this offers further support to the view that personal judgement is a highly sensitive – even hair trigger – process.

6. So much about how we decide remains mysterious. Over the last 80 years or so, human judgement has been the subject of sustained investigation by psychologists, neuroscientists, economic theorists and philosophers. Yet despite learning much about common errors and biases in decision-making, nearly a century of scientific research has told us more about what we don't know than we do, including:

   ... (1) human cognition is not under our control, (2) we are not aware of our judgement and decision processes and (3) our reports of those processes are not to be trusted ... **(26)**

7. That said, we think there are six central facts about personal judgement which we should acknowledge:

   FACT ONE: NURSING AND HEALTHCARE DECISION-MAKING IS MOSTLY GREY

   FACT TWO: WE DO NOT STAND APART FROM THE WORLD AROUND US

   FACT THREE: IT'S IMPOSSIBLE TO CARE IN A FULLY DETACHED MANNER

   FACT FOUR: MEMBERSHIP OF A PROFESSION NO MORE GUARANTEES AGREED DECISION-MAKING THAN MEMBERSHIP OF A FAMILY DOES

   FACT FIVE: ETHICAL DECISION-MAKING IS NOT LIKE EVIDENCE-BASED PRACTICE

   FACT SIX: ETHICAL CODES ALWAYS REQUIRE PERSONAL INTERPRETATION

8. According to Nobel Prize-winning psychological research we 'think fast' rather than reflect carefully for the great majority of our decisions. We believe, but cannot yet prove, that this applies to many ethical judgements too.

9. From the extensive literature on the psychology of decision-making, we know that in reality health professionals simply do not make their decisions 'according to the book' – rather, they make them as dynamic, extraordinarily complex, human beings.

10. Nursing practice is not carried out by neutral individuals, far from it. Nursing, healthcare and life in general is like the complex **Train Journey** we describe in **Chapter Three**, concluding:

   There are no protocols and no definitive ethical guidance for life's train journeys. There are no neutral experiences on the train. The passengers are not separate from the journey's events. They affect the events and the events affect them. Precisely how this will happen is always unpredictable, for any journey.

11. All this, and much more in the body of the book, calls much of our existing practice and education into question. There is value in policies and codes, but these must always be placed in context and must always be implemented by people – who inevitably will make their own judgements about how best to do this.

This is slowly coming to be acknowledged by official bodies, including the **NMC** who say, when considering nurses' 'fitness to practise':

> We think it's important that we work more closely with employers so that as many issues as possible can be resolved quickly and effectively at a local level. We'll give more consideration to the context in which incidents occur, in recognition of the complex issues and unique pressures nurses and midwives face every day in the NHS. **(176)**

And:

> ... there is limited understanding of the consequences of working with different contexts. **(177)**

12. After much consideration of these complexities, we continue to assert the importance of personal judgement in nursing and beyond. In the end, all judgement is personal.
13. We also believe that it is only through developing a deeper appreciation of the true role of personal judgement that we will bring about better care. The best method we can think of at the moment is to evolve healthcare education to include the factors we identify in this book – and no doubt many more – and to have the resolve to address the variabilities and uncertainties of life realistically, seriously and extensively.
14. One of the most effective ways to do this – possibly the most effective – is to encourage repeated practice in real life or simulated real-life decision-making, always drawing attention to the ways in which we are all – professionals and patients – influenced and changeable.

CONCLUSION: THE SPECTRA ARE MYTHS TOO

In this book we've presented three different spectra to illustrate a central tension in nursing and healthcare. Few dispute that a 'check-box' culture has evolved in recent years, and that this has begun to erode and devalue personal judgement, and we needed a simple way to depict this, in relation to autonomous decision-making.

We've used the left-hand poles to epitomise fixed rules and standards, step-by-step decision-making, consistency and conformity, while we've made the right-hand poles represent creativity, personal involvement and choice. We've used this technique in order to help nurses and health carers contemplate where on the spectra they have chosen to sit, or where they are being asked to sit by their employers.

We were tempted to include a further spectrum in the book's conclusion, in the same vein, with uniformity at the left and autonomy to the right. However, we came to realise that this would, ironically, be to fall into exactly the mindset we're trying to discourage, despite our disclaimers dotted about the book. To think about the world in 'either/or' terms is over-simplistic. It's like saying some of the passengers on the **Train Journey** are able to think for themselves, while others are robotic and incapable of independent thought: a false and potentially insulting idea, which we do not believe but which we could be judged to be perpetuating, if we did not explain ourselves sufficiently clearly.

We're aware that we're in danger of allowing a very basic, illustrative model to appear to be the entire reality, which it most definitely is not.

We've almost fallen into the trap of believing our own simplistic framing.

There's no doubt that the left and right poles represent a palpable tension in nursing and healthcare, and that this tension has real-life effects on a daily basis. But – just like the other myths we describe in **Chapter Three** – it can be counterbalanced by a deeper, richer reality that offers the hope of an increasingly creative, personal healthcare environment. Autonomy and standardisation can be and often are at odds, yet it's naive to suggest that one or the other has to be the ultimate rationale for nursing and healthcare.

We're not alone in seeing a split between obeying the rules and making free choices. It's everywhere in the literature. For example, when discussing professionalism the **NMC** states prominently that:

> Professionalism is characterised by the **autonomous** evidence-based deci-sion making by members of an occupation who SHARE THE SAME VALUES and education.

It also states:

> The ultimate purpose of professionalism in nursing and midwifery is to ensure the CONSISTENT provision of SAFE, EFFECTIVE, **person-centred** outcomes ... [which] can be demonstrated through ... **individualised** care and services evidenced through support for **personal choices** and increased involvement in decision mak-ing about planned care or services. **(178)** (bold and capitals ours, to illustrate the naive dichotomy)

From a strictly philosophical point of view this is contradictory. Seen naively, if you share the same values as everyone else you will decide in the same way as everyone else and so autonomy is irrelevant. And if you set out to be consistent and safe then being person-centred is irrelevant, since you will always act in the same, safe ways regardless of what the person you are caring for wants. But the strictly philosophical view is unreal: **the apparent dichotomies are instantly resolved once personal judgement is properly understood.**

The polarised concepts can seem totally opposed, but serious reflection on how we decide in real-life contexts shows a more profound picture, revealed by reflection on any of the scenarios. Our spectra do not exist in any solid way. Rather, the poles – and everything in between – should be seen as options, to be used as judged fit, by personal decision-makers.

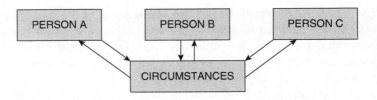

Figure 8.13   Different People and Different Circumstances

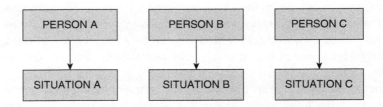

Figure 8.14   The Person Plus the Circumstances Create Different Situations

When personal judgement occurs, the person can choose the approach or combination of approaches regardless of where they sit on the spectra to create a plan (consciously or unconsciously) and to act:

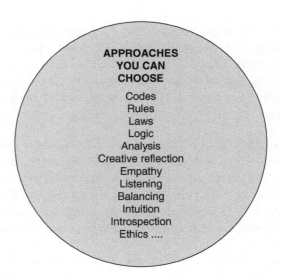

Figure 8.15   Choosing the Appropriate Approach

Any of the options – to the left or right of the spectra – can be chosen. It's up to the decision-maker to use her judgement to choose which is best in the circumstances: fixed rules or fluid thinking. It's up to the person deciding.

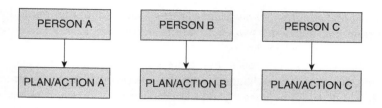

Figure 8.16   Planning and Acting

The spectra dissolve because personal judgement is always primary. This is a fact of human life. Whether to follow an exact protocol or dismiss it and try something altogether different is up to the person, up to the healthcare: it's up to you.

No one sits permanently to the left or right – you can decide what approach to use, and whatever you use it does not commit you to the left or the right for every decision. The most maverick nurse can choose tried and trusted approaches – or to apply a well-known ethical principle – if she judges that this will be best. And the most conformist, rule-abiding practitioner is perpetually free to go against policy if she has good reasons to do so.

The default in nursing and healthcare at present is the left of the spectrum – if you are a habitual rule follower that is where you will be. But you need to be constantly aware that this is a choice, and you can change it. It's simply false to think you have no choice, that you have to go along with the status quo, that your professional role is 'just to obey orders'. You're a person and so you're massively more complex, inventive and important than that. You always have a choice, and the more you practise choosing, and the more you picture yourself and others as you work, the more you will be self-aware, creative and flexible in your judgements.

Personal judgement is the primary force in nursing and healthcare. Using it dissolves spectra and unhelpful dichotomies. It breaks down barriers and frees you to be yourself and a true professional at the same time, able to offer thoughtful, effective healthcare to everyone you encounter.

And even if this is not what you want, you can't escape the responsibility, so you may as well embrace it and all it offers.

WHAT IF I GO AGAINST THE RULES AND MAKE A BAD DECISION?

Finally, we do understand that many people – both students and experienced health professionals – may feel anxious and unnerved by the position we have presented in this book. We are very aware that it may seem much easier and safer simply to 'obey the law' or 'follow the code' or 'do what it says in the manual'. And this is indeed a choice.

The problem is that this is just one choice out of many options, and it's no safer than any other. As we've seen so extensively, everything in life is open to interpretation – including the meaning and relevance of laws, codes and policies – and, therefore, the personal element cannot be avoided. As we quote at the start of the book: if you choose not to decide you still have made a choice.

Rather than cling to a false belief that there are, somewhere, books and papers and declarations that can tell you what to do with absolute certainty, it's surely far better to be realistic, to accept that sometimes you will make decisions that not everyone will agree with, and that you will need to be able to justify these. It's surely far better to try to understand yourself and the complexities of life and other people – to realise that yes, sometimes you may 'get it wrong' – than vainly seek a mythical Holy Grail of decision-making.

HOW DOES THIS BOOK HELP YOU?

We can understand that it may seem that by introducing the many complexities of personal judgement, and by pointing out that you simply have to use personal judgement in healthcare decision-making, we have made matters worse for readers looking for clear and simple guidance. However, we believe that acknowledging the reality is the only meaningful option available, and that with practice and informed reflection, awareness and expertise will grow. This does not mean that you will make more and more correct judgements, since so much in this area is open to debate, but it will help you:

GAIN CONFIDENCE IN YOUR DECISION-MAKING AND JUDGEMENTS

Because it is apparent that all your decisions depend on you, in whatever circumstances prevail, rather than on some external command (if you are commanded you still need to decide whether to obey), you will gain confidence as you assert your independence. You will not always make ideal decisions (if such things exist) but you will have full ownership of your choices and will, therefore, learn more readily than if you believe you are merely following the rules.

BECOME MORE ACCOUNTABLE AND ABLE TO JUSTIFY YOURSELF AS AN AUTONOMOUS PRACTITIONER

Routinely writing out why you made your judgements is an invaluable way to present evidence of your decision-making reasoning and process. You may not always know exactly why you chose as you did, but taking the trouble to understand and explain, even if only to yourself, will increasingly empower you and prepare you to deal with any challenges to your judgements that will inevitably arise in your work.

PROTECT YOURSELF FROM TRUST, NMC OR LEGAL ACTIONS AGAINST YOU

If you can habitually provide not only factual evidence and evidence from the literature to support your judgements, but also explain how you understood the unique situation you encountered as a human being, referring to **PSP PLUS** if you wish, then you will be very much better protected from any formal actions than if you are less overtly aware.

BE BETTER ABLE TO SATISFY REVALIDATION REQUIREMENTS

Amongst much else, the current **NMC** revalidation process asks nurses to apply both the **6Cs** and the **NMC** code to reflections about practice. Knowing more about the real nature of personal judgement will help you understand and explain that both approaches are limited in what they can do, and are just two amongst many alternatives. You will be able to explain where interpretation is necessary – as it surely is – and to say why and how you have added your personal judgement to the reflections, in a mature, knowledgeable and self-aware fashion.

CHAPTER EIGHT EXERCISES

Having read **Chapter Eight** you may like to attempt the following exercises, to reinforce your learning:

1. Choose a scenario from **Chapters Five, Six** or **Seven** and apply the **Rings of Uncertainty** to it
2. Express the **Rings** for yourself
3. Express the **Rings** for another person – real or imagined – who takes a different view from you
4. Write a short essay describing an imaginary 'train journey' of your own. It need not be an actual train journey. It can be any 'life journey" involving yourself, other people and their interactions.

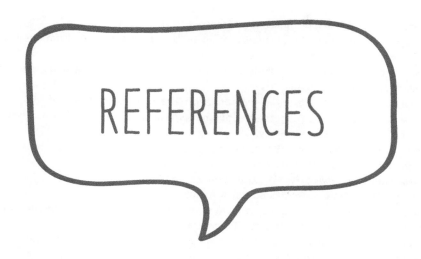

REFERENCES

1. Standing, M. (2017). *Clinical Judgement and Decision Making in Nursing* (Transforming Nursing Practice Series), 3rd edn. London: Sage.
2. Benner, P. (1999). Nursing leadership for the new millennium. Claiming the wisdom & worth of clinical practice. *Nurse Health Care Perspective. 20*(6):312–19.
3. Hedberg, B. & Larsson, U.S. (2003). Observations, confirmations and strategies – useful tools in decision-making process for nurses in practice? *Journal of Clinical Nursing. 12*(2):215–22.
4. Cioffi 2009 (https://sigmapubs.onlinelibrary.wiley.com/doi/full/10.1111/j.1741-6787.2008.00138.x)
5. www.nmc.org.uk/globalassets/sitedocuments/other-publications/enabling-professionalism.pdf
6. Darbyshire, P. (2017) 'Intentional Rounding' – the best intentions or is nursing being dumbed-down?, *Ausmed*, 18 June, www.ausmed.com/cpd/articles/intentional-rounding [Accessed 16 Aug. 2019]
7. Forde-Johnston, C. (2014) *Intentional rounding: a review of the literature.* [online] Rcni.com. Available at: http://journals.rcni.com/nursing-standard/intentional-rounding-a-review-of-the-literature-ns2014.04.28.32.37.e8564 [Accessed 16 Aug. 2019]
8. www.rt.com/news/hospital-cover-up-uk-190/ [Accessed 16 Aug. 2019]
9. www.dailymail.co.uk/health/article-5438429/Government-announces-review-three-health-scandals.html [Accessed 16 Aug. 2019]
10. www.itv.com/news/2013-02-06/key-recommendations-of-nhs-mid-staffordshire-public-inquiry/ [Accessed 16 Aug. 2019]
11. www.theguardian.com/society/2012/jan/06/nurses-hourly-rounds-cameron-hospitals [Accessed 16 Aug. 2019]
12. www.theguardian.com/society/2018/feb/02/nhs-compensation-payouts-unsustainable-say-health-leaders [Accessed 16 Aug. 2019]
13. https://rcni.com/revalidation/6cs-of-nursing-32156 [Accessed 16 Aug. 2019]
14. www.nmc.org.uk/globalassets/sitedocuments/education-standards/future-nurse-proficiencies.pdf [Accessed 16 Aug. 2019]
15. www.nmc.org.uk/standards/standards-for-nurses/ [Accessed 16 Aug. 2019]
16. www.nmc.org.uk/standards/standards-for-nurses/pre-2018-standards/ [Accessed 16 Aug. 2019]

17. www.nmc.org.uk/standards/guidance/ [Accessed 16 Aug. 2019]
18. www.nmc.org.uk/standards/standards-for-nurses/standards-for-pre-registration-nursing-programmes/ [Accessed 16 Aug. 2019]
19. www.nmc.org.uk/globalassets/sitedocuments/education-standards/programme-standards-nursing.pdf [Accessed 16 Aug. 2019]
20. Seedhouse, D.F. (2009) *Ethics: the Heart of Health Care*. Chichester: Wiley, 3rd edn.
21. www.nmc.org.uk/globalassets/sitedocuments/education-standards/future-nurse-proficiencies.pdf [Accessed 16 Aug. 2019]
22. https://en.wikipedia.org/wiki/Bystander_effect [Accessed 16 Aug. 2019]
23. www.youtube.com/watch?v=OSsPfbup0ac [Accessed 16 Aug. 2019]
24. www.youtube.com/watch?v=z4S1LLrSzVE [Accessed 16 Aug. 2019]
25. Lehrer, J. (2009) *How we Decide*. Boston, MA: Houghton Mifflin Harcourt.
26. Hammond, Kenneth, R. (1996) *Human Judgment and Social Policy: Irreducible Uncertainty, Inevitable Error, Unavoidable Injustice*. Oxford University Press USA.
27. https://suebehaviouraldesign.com/kahneman-fast-slow-thinking/ [Accessed 16 Aug. 2019]
28. www.nmc.org.uk/standards/code/read-the-code-online/ [Accessed 16 Aug. 2019]
29. www.youtube.com/watch?v=PirFrDVRBo4 [Accessed 16 Aug. 2019]
30. http://currentnursing.com/theory/decision_making_models.html [Accessed 16 Aug. 2019]
31. www.bon.texas.gov/pdfs/delegation_pdfs/School%20Nurse%20Delegation%20Decision%20Trees.pdf [Accessed 16 Aug. 2019]
32. www.ncsbn.org/Clinical_Judgment_Lit_Review_Executive_Summary.pdf [Accessed 16 Aug. 2019]
33. Ida Torunn Bjørk and Glenys A. Hamilton, Clinical decision making of nurses working in hospital settings, *Nursing Research and Practice*, Volume *2011* (www.hindawi.com/journals/nrp/2011/524918/) [Accessed 16 Aug. 2019]
34. www.ncbi.nlm.nih.gov/pmc/articles/PMC2893088/ [Accessed 16 Aug. 2019]
35. https://journals.lww.com/nursingmadeincrediblyeasy/fulltext/2015/11000/The_pathway_to_best_practice.13.aspx [Accessed 16 Aug. 2019]
36. www.nursingprocess.org/Nursing-Process-Steps.html [Accessed 16 Aug. 2019]
37. https://en.wikipedia.org/wiki/Nursing_process [Accessed 16 Aug. 2019]
38. www.ncbi.nlm.nih.gov/pmc/articles/PMC4525336/ [Accessed 16 Aug. 2019]
39. www.researchgate.net/figure/The-nursing-knowledge-and-decision-making-model-McCloskey-and-Bulechek-1992-adapted-by_fig2_283092035 [Accessed 16 Aug. 2019]
40. https://flowpsychology.com/10-humanistic-approach-strengths-and-weaknesses/ [Accessed 16 Aug. 2019]
41. Seedhouse, D.F (2000) *Practical Nursing Philosophy*. Chichester: Wiley.
42. Knowlden, V. (1990) The virtue of caring in nursing. In Madeleine M. Leininger (ed.) *Ethical and Moral Dimensions of Care*. Detroit: Wayne State University Press.
43. www.brookes.ac.uk/students/upgrade/study-skills/reflective-writing-gibbs/ [Accessed 16 Aug. 2019]
44. Mayeroff, M. (1971) *On Caring*. London: Harper and Row.
45. Curtin, L. (1986) The Nurse as Advocate: A philosophical foundation for nursing. In Peggy. L. Chinn (ed.) *Ethical Issues in Nursing*. Maryland: Aspen Systems Corporation.
46. Gadow, S. (1983) Existential advocacy: philosophical foundation of nursing. In C.P. Murphy and H. Hunter (eds.) *Ethical Problems in the Nurse–patient Relationship*. Boston, MA: Allyn & Bacon, pp 40–58.
47. https://journals.lww.com/nursing/fulltext/2015/03000/The_Roper_Logan_Tierney_model_of_nursing__A.9.aspx [Accessed 16 Aug. 2019]

48. www.datadictionary.nhs.uk/data_dictionary/attributes/a/a_and_e_initial_assessment_triage_category_de.asp?shownav=1 [Accessed 16 Aug. 2019]

49. Thompson, C., Cullum, N., McCaughan, D., Sheldon, T. and Raynor, P. (2004) Nurses, information use, and clinical decision making – the real world potential for evidence-based decisions in nursing. *Evidence-based Nursing*, Vol. 7, 3.

50. www.sign.ac.uk/sign-158-british-guideline-on-the-management-of-asthma.html see pages 85–88 [Accessed 16 Aug. 2019]

51. www.investopedia.com/terms/c/cost-benefitanalysis.asp [Accessed 16 Aug. 2019]

52. www.investopedia.com/ask/answers/040315/what-difference-between-risk-avoidance-and-risk-reduction.asp [Accessed 16 Aug. 2019]

53. www.investopedia.com/ask/answers/040315/what-difference-between-risk-avoidance-and-risk-reduction.asp [Accessed 16 Aug. 2019]

54. Fulford, K.W.M., Peile, Ed, Carroll, Heidi (2012) *Essential Values-Based Practice*. Cambridge: CUP.

55. https://onlinelibrary.wiley.com/doi/10.1002/9780470510544.ch1 [Accessed 16 Aug. 2019]

56. https://vxcommunity.com [Accessed 16 Aug. 2019]

57. www.scottishlegal.com/article/blanket-ban-smoking-mental-health-hospitals-declared-lawful [Accessed 16 Aug. 2019]

58. www.itv.com/news/central/2016-05-11/e-cigarettes-allowed-on-hospital-grounds-after-policy-change/ [Accessed 16 Aug. 2019]

59. www.gov.uk/government/publications/e-cigarettes-and-heated-tobacco-products-evidence-review/evidence-review-of-e-cigarettes-and-heated-tobacco-products-2018-executive-summary [Accessed 16 Aug. 2019]

60. https://publichealthmatters.blog.gov.uk/2018/02/20/clearing-up-some-myths-around-e-cigarettes/ [Accessed 16 Aug. 2019]

61. www.itv.com/news/central/2016-05-11/e-cigarettes-allowed-on-hospital-grounds-after-policy-change/ [Accessed 16 Aug. 2019]

62. https://expertvaping.com/uk-hospitals-lift-vaping-ban/ [Accessed 16 Aug. 2019]

63. www.legislation.gov.uk/ukpga/2010/15/section/15 [Accessed 16 Aug. 2019]

64. www.gazettelive.co.uk/news/teesside-news/please-dont-smoke-hospital-entrances-9898854 [Accessed 16 Aug. 2019]

65. http://condoadviser.ca/2016/02/condominiums-can-prevent-smoking-in-units/condo-law-blog-Ontario [Accessed 16 Aug. 2019]

66. www.cancer.net/navigating-cancer-care/prevention-and-healthy-living/stopping-tobacco-use-after-cancer-diagnosis/health-risks-e-cigarettes-smokeless-tobacco-and-waterpipes [Accessed 16 Aug. 2019]

67. www.dummies.com/careers/project-management/performing-a-cost-benefit-analysis/ [Accessed 16 Aug. 2019]

68. www.smartsheet.com/expert-guide-cost-benefit-analysis [Accessed 16 Aug. 2019]

69. Seedhouse, D.F. (2107) *Thoughtful Health Care*. London: Sage.

70. www.dailymail.co.uk/news/article-2591250/Flowers-ban-9-10-hospitals-concerns-blooms-spread-germs.html#ixzz3vuMnFYmT [Accessed 16 Aug. 2019]

71. www.americanscientist.org/article/understanding-the-butterfly-effect

72. Buchanan, A., (2011) *Better than Human*. Oxford: Oxford University Press.

73. www.nurse.com/evidence-based-practice [Accessed 16 Aug. 2019]

74. https://doi.org/10.1016/j.lungcan.2016.05.011 [Accessed 16 Aug. 2019]

75. https://publichealthmatters.blog.gov.uk/2018/02/19/creating-a-smokefree-nhs-how-e-cigarettes-can-help/ [Accessed 16 Aug. 2019]

76. www.lungcancernews.org/2017/04/01/should-physicians-recommend-e-cigarettes-to-their-lung-cancer-patients-who-smoke-what-about-their-family-members-... [Accessed 16 Aug. 2019]

77. https://scienceblog.cancerresearchuk.org/2017/02/06/new-study-comes-the-closest-yet-to-proving-that-e-cigarettes-arent-as-dangerous-as-smoking/ [Accessed 16 Aug. 2019]

78. https://publichealthmatters.blog.gov.uk/2018/02/20/clearing-up-some-myths-around-e-cigarettes/ [Accessed 16 Aug. 2019]

79. http://otresearch.vxcommunity.com [Accessed 16 Aug. 2019]

80. https://journals.sagepub.com/doi/full/10.1177/0308022619829722 [Accessed 16 Aug. 2019]

81. McShea, M.M (1978) Clinical judgment: an ethical issue. *J Psychiatr Nurs Ment Health Serv.*, Mar; *16*(3): 52–5. www.ncbi.nlm.nih.gov/pubmed/213575 [Accessed 16 Aug. 2019]

82. www.ukcen.net/ethical_issues/ethical_frameworks/the_four_principles_of_biomedical_ethics [Accessed 16 Aug. 2019]

83. https://jme.bmj.com/content/37/10/582.full [Accessed 16 Aug. 2019]

84. www.ncbi.nlm.nih.gov/pmc/articles/PMC3528420/ [Accessed 16 Aug. 2019]

85. http://blogs.biomedcentral.com/bmcseriesblog/2012/07/13/measuring-the-four-principles-of-beauchamp-and-childress/ [Accessed 16 Aug. 2019]

86. Fry, S.T., Veatch, R.M. and Taylor, C.R. (2010) *Case Studies in Nursing Ethics*, 4th edn. Burlington, MA: Jones & Bartlett Publishers.

87. Thompson, I., Melia, K., Boyd, K. and Horsburgh, D. (2006) *Nursing Ethics*, 6th edn. London: Churchill Livingstone.

88. www.sciencedaily.com/releases/2008/03/080305144210.htm [Accessed 16 Aug. 2019]

89. Hodgkinson, G.P., Langan-Fox, J. and Sadler-Smith, E. (2008) Intuition: A fundamental bridging construct in the behavioural sciences. *British Journal of Psychology*, *99*: 1–27.

90. Hams, S.P. (2000) A gut feeling? *Intuition and Critical Care Nursing*, *16*(5): 310–18.

91. Kahneman, D. (2012) *Thinking, Fast and Slow*. London: Penguin.

92. Klein, G. (1999) *Sources of Power: How People Make Decisions*. Cambridge, MA: MIT Press.

93. Polanyi, M. *Personal Knowledge*. University Of Chicago Press; Corr. (15 August 1974).

94. www.ncbi.nlm.nih.gov/pmc/articles/PMC3325865/ [Accessed 16 Aug. 2019]

95. http://currentnursing.com/nursing_theory/Patricia_Benner_From_Novice_to_Expert.html [Accessed 16 Aug. 2019]

96. www.sciencedirect.com/science/article/abs/pii/S0884217517304045 [Accessed 16 Aug. 2019]

97. www.ncbi.nlm.nih.gov/m/pubmed/11000605/ [Accessed 16 Aug. 2019]

98. www.opastonline.com/wp-content/uploads/2016/12/intuition-an-important-tool-in-the-practice-of-nursing-jnh-16-014.pdf [Accessed 16 Aug. 2019]

99. www.researchgate.net/publication/253650486_Intuition_in_Nursing_Practice [Accessed 16 Aug. 2019]

100. https://thenextweb.com/contributors/2018/11/03/our-lack-of-interest-in-data-ethics-will-come-back-to-haunt-us/amp/ [Accessed 16 Aug. 2019]

101. www.dailymotion.com/video/x3q4alx [Accessed 16 Aug. 2019]

102. www.psychologytoday.com/articles/200705/intuition-heads-in-the-clouds [Accessed 16 Aug. 2019]

103. https://onlinelibrary.wiley.com/doi/abs/10.1111/j.1466-769X.2011.00507.x [Accessed 16 Aug. 2019]

104. www.researchgate.net/profile/Rob_Pooley/publication/267232065/figure/fig1/AS:295681316147205@1447507327641/Ethical-Grid-Seedhouse-1998.png [Accessed 16 Aug. 2019]

105. www.danalbrightmd.com/blog/what-are-the-three-approaches-for-total-hip-replacement-surgery-1536/ [Accessed 16 Aug. 2019]

106. Carr, S.M., Bell, B., Pearson, P.H. and Watson, D.W. (2001) To be sure or not to be sure: Concepts of uncertainty and risk in the construction of community nursing practice. *Primary Health Care Research and Development*, 2: 223–33

107. Cioffi, J. (1998) Decision-making by emergency nurses in triage assessments. *Accident and Emergency Nursing*, 6: 184–91.

108. www.simplypsychology.org/milgram.html [Accessed 16 Aug. 2019]

109. www.simplypsychology.org/zimbardo.html [Accessed 16 Aug. 2019]

110. Ballat, J. and Campling, P. (2011) *Intelligent Kindness: Reforming the culture of healthcare*. RCPsych Publications.

111. Damasio, A. (1994) *Descartes Error*. New York: Grosset/Putnam.

112. www.psychologytoday.com/us/basics/emotional-intelligence [Accessed 16 Aug. 2019]

113. www.researchgate.net/publication/281214332_Values-based_practice_Translating_values_and_evidence_into_good_clinical_care [Accessed 16 Aug. 2019]

114. www.ncbi.nlm.nih.gov/pmc/articles/PMC2587197/

115. Peile, Ed (2014) Teaching balanced clinical decision-making in primary care: evidence-based and values-based approaches used in conjunction. *Educ Prim Care*, 25(2): 67–70.

116. www.nursingtimes.net/would-you-stop-to-provide-care/1866313.article [Accessed 16 Aug. 2019]

117. https://nurse.org/articles/off-duty-nursing-dilemma/ [Accessed 16 Aug. 2019]

118. https://nurse.org/articles/off-duty-nursing-dilemma/ [Accessed 16 Aug. 2019]

119. https://www.youtube.com/watch?v=BzMl_yzcaxo [Accessed 16 Aug. 2019]

120. https://en.wikipedia.org/wiki/The_Vocation_of_Man [Accessed 16 Aug. 2019]

121. Ariely, D. (2009) *Predictably Irrational*. Harper Collins.

122. https://en.wikipedia.org/wiki/List_of_cognitive_biases [Accessed 16 Aug. 2019]

123. www.reference.com/world-view/examples-personal-biases-a54b58cca11f2b82, www.psychologytoday.com/us/basics/bias [Accessed 16 Aug. 2019]

124. www.fastcompany.com/90303107/how-to-become-a-less-biased-version-of-yourself [Accessed 16 Aug. 2019]

125. Hollnagel, E. (2017) *Safety in Practice: Developing the Resilience Potentials*. Taylor and Francis.

126. Argyle, M. (1994) *The Psychology of Interpersonal Behaviour*, 5th edn. Penguin.

127. https://journals.sagepub.com/doi/abs/10.1177/0956797618822697?journalCode=pssa [Accessed 16 Aug. 2019]

128. www.theguardian.com/commentisfree/2017/feb/19/think-empathy-makes-world-better-place-think-again [Accessed 16 Aug. 2019]

129. www.bmj.com/content/340/bmj.c1478 [Accessed 16 Aug. 2019]

130. http://news.bbc.co.uk/1/hi/health/8570866.stm [Accessed 16 Aug. 2019]

131. www.england.nhs.uk/wp-content/uploads/2016/05/cip-yr-3.pdf [Accessed 16 Aug. 2019]

132. https://improvement.nhs.uk/resources/healthcare-associated-infections [Accessed 16 Aug. 2019]

133. www.lawyers.com/legal-info/criminal/criminal-law-basics/reporting-crimes-witnessing-ignoring-falsely-reporting-and-lying.html/ [Accessed 16 Aug. 2019]

134. www.rcpch.ac.uk/resources/pre-procedure-pregnancy-checking-under-16s-clinical-guideline

135. Mental Capacity Act, 2005

136. Coffey, M. and Byrt, R. (2010) *Forensic Mental Health Nursing. Ethics, Debates and Dilemmas*. London: Quay Books.
137. Mayer, J.D. and Salovey, P. (1997) What is emotional intelligence? In P. Salovey and D.J. Sluyter (eds), *Emotional Development and Emotional Intelligence: Implications for educators*. New York: Basic Books.
138. Mental Health Act, 1983
139. www.cqc.org.uk/guidance-providers/regulations-enforcement/regulation-20-duty-candour [Accessed 16 Aug. 2019]
140. Medicines Act, 1968
141. www.nursingtimes.net/clinical-archive/patient-safety/the-12-hour-shift-friend-or-foe/5081694.article [Accessed 16 Aug. 2019]
142. www.rcn.org.uk/professional-development/publications/PUB-006051 [Accessed 16 Aug. 2019]
143. www.cancer.org/cancer/testicular-cancer/detection-diagnosis-staging/survival-rates.html [Accessed 16 Aug. 2019]
144. www.dbth.nhs.uk/wp-content/uploads/2017/10/Guidelines-for-Administration-of-Naloxone.pdf [Accessed 16 Aug. 2019]
145. www.healthcareers.nhs.uk/working-health/making-every-contact-count [Accessed 16 Aug. 2019]
146. www.crisisprevention.com/Blog/September-2011/Domestic-Violence-What-Can-Nurses-Do [Accessed 16 Aug. 2019]
147. www.ncbi.nlm.nih.gov/pmc/articles/PMC196400/ [Accessed 16 Aug. 2019]
148. www.rcn.org.uk/clinical-topics/domestic-violence-and-abuse/professional-resources [Accessed 16 Aug. 2019]
149. www.healthcareers.nhs.uk/working-health/making-every-contact-count [Accessed 16 Aug. 2019]
150. www.crisisprevention.com/Blog/September-2011/Domestic-Violence-What-Can-Nurses-Do [Accessed 16 Aug. 2019]
151. www.cdc.gov/vaccines/hcp/vis/vis-statements/mmr.html [Accessed 16 Aug. 2019]
152. https://assets.publishing.service.gov.uk/government/uploads/system/uploads/attachment_data/file/663453/Reducing_the_Need_for_Restraint_and_Restrictive_Intervention.pdf [Accessed 16 Aug. 2019]
153. www.legislation.gov.uk/ukpga/2010/15/introduction [Accessed 16 Aug. 2019]
154. www.legislation.gov.uk/ukpga/2005/9/pdfs/ukpgacop_20050009_en.pdf [Accessed 16 Aug. 2019]
155. www.legislation.gov.uk/ukpga/2005/9/resources [Accessed 16 Aug. 2019]
156. https://emedicine.medscape.com/article/1156220-overview [Accessed 16 Aug. 2019]
157. https://cks.nice.org.uk/falls-risk-assessment [Accessed 16 Aug. 2019]
158. www.healthline.com/health/schizophrenia/alternative-treatments [Accessed 16 Aug. 2019]
159. www.all-about-psychology.com/the-myth-of-mental-illness.html [Accessed 16 Aug. 2019]
160. https://breggin.com/toxic-psychiatry/ [Accessed 16 Aug. 2019]
161. www.psychiatry.org/psychiatrists/practice/dsm [Accessed 16 Aug. 2019]
162. www.rethink.org/living-with-mental-illness/police-courts-prison/section-37-hospital-order [Accessed 16 Aug. 2019]
163. www.abc.net.au/radionational/programs/philosopherszone/the-philosophy-of-compassion/3438182#transcript [Accessed 16 Aug. 2019]
164. www.ncbi.nlm.nih.gov/pubmed/21378657 [Accessed 16 Aug. 2019]

165. www.nhs.uk/conditions/consent-to-treatment/children/ [Accessed 16 Aug. 2019]

166. www.gmc-uk.org/ethical-guidance/ethical-guidance-for-doctors/0-18-years/principles-of-confidentiality [Accessed 16 Aug. 2019]

167. www.fastcompany.com/3038060/3-ways-to-improve-your-personal-judgement [Accessed 16 Aug. 2019]

168. www.pointofcarefoundation.org.uk/our-work/ [Accessed 16 Aug. 2019]

169. www.youtube.com/watch?time_continue=79&v=--uMNY55nw4 [Accessed 16 Aug. 2019]

170. www.pointofcarefoundation.org.uk/resource/patient-family-centred-care-toolkit/tools/patient-family-centred-care-tools-overview/ [Accessed 16 Aug. 2019]

171. www.pointofcarefoundation.org.uk/our-work/sweeney-programme/about-the-sweeney-programme/ [Accessed 16 Aug. 2019]

172. www.pointofcarefoundation.org.uk/our-work/sweeney-programme/sweeney-methodology/ [Accessed 16 Aug. 2019]

173. www.pointofcarefoundation.org.uk/evidence-resources/ [Accessed 16 Aug. 2019]

174. www.wikihow.com/Make-Better-Decisions [Accessed 16 Aug. 2019]

175. Seedhouse, D.F. (1991) *Liberating Medicine*. Chichester: Wiley

176. www.nmc.org.uk/concerns-nurses-midwives/fitness-to-practise-a-new-approach/ [Accessed 16 Aug. 2019]

177. www.ncbi.nlm.nih.gov/m/pubmed/11895535/ [Accessed 16 Aug. 2019]

178. www.nmc.org.uk/globalassets/sitedocuments/other-publications/enabling-professionalism.pdf [Accessed 16 Aug. 2019]

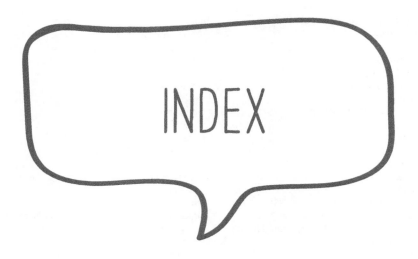

INDEX